Atlas of Infrared Spectra of Drugs

药 品 红 外 光 谱 集

第五卷（2015）

国家药典委员会　编

中国医药科技出版社

图书在版编目（CIP）数据

药品红外光谱集. 第 5 卷. 2015/国家药典委员会编.
—北京：中国医药科技出版社，2015.8
ISBN 978 - 7 - 5067 - 7700 - 1

Ⅰ. ①药… Ⅱ. ①国… Ⅲ. ①药品检定—红外分光光
度法—图谱 Ⅳ. ①R927. 11 - 64

中国版本图书馆 CIP 数据核字（2015）第 148724 号

ISBN 978-7-5067-7700-1

责任编辑
美术编辑

出版　中国医药科技出版社
地址　北京市海淀区文慧园北路甲 22 号
邮编　100082
电话　发行：010 - 62227427　邮购：010 - 62236938
网址　www. cmstp. com
规格　889 × 1194mm $^1/_{16}$
印张　10
字数　229 千字
版次　2015 年 8 月第 1 版
印次　2015 年 8 月第 1 次印刷
印刷　三河市万龙印装有限公司
经销　全国各地新华书店
书号　978 - 7 - 5067 - 7700 - 1
定价　198. 00 元

本社图书如存在印装质量问题请与本社联系调换

《药品红外光谱集》第五卷（2015）编委会名单

主　　编　凌大奎　王　平

副 主 编　李慧义　王　绯

编　　委（按姓氏笔画排序）

王　平　　王　绯　　厉进忠　　白政忠　　刘　敏　　刘英慧　　李　琦

李文莉　　李昌亮　　李晓东　　李珺婵　　李慧义　　吴　燕　　余振喜

张立雯　　张雅军　　陈民辉　　武向峰　　范婷婷　　郑国钢　　胡　敏

姜连阁　　董朝瑜　　楼永军　　阚家义

目　　录

前言

说明

聚苯乙烯薄膜标准红外光谱图

药品红外光谱图 ·· 光谱号 1229

中文名索引 ·· 索引 1 ～ 3

英文名索引 ·· 索引 5 ～ 7

分子式索引 ·· 索引 9 ～ 11

中文名总索引 ·· 索引 13 ～ 30

英文名总索引 ·· 索引 31 ～ 48

前　　言

　　红外光谱法是有机化合物分析中广泛应用的方法。由于红外光谱的高度专属性，在药品检验中，红外光谱法常与其他理化方法联合使用，作为有机药品重要的鉴别方法。鉴于有机药品品种不断增加，特别是许多药品化学结构比较复杂或相互之间化学结构差异较小，当用颜色反应、沉淀、结晶形成或紫外-可见分光光度法等常用方法不足以相互区分时，红外光谱法更是行之有效的鉴别手段。

　　《中华人民共和国药典》（二部）自1977年版开始采用红外光谱法用于一些药品的鉴别，在该版药典附录中收载了对照图谱。为了适应我国对药品监督检验的需要，1985年，国家药典委员会委托部分省、市药品检验所收集绘制了国产药品红外光谱图423幅，编制出版了《药品红外光谱集》1985年版，作为药品鉴别用红外对照图谱。鉴于《中华人民共和国药典》及国家药品标准均收载红外光谱法，应用红外光谱鉴别的品种不断增加，有必要在原有基础上扩大收载范围，为此，国家药典委员会正式组织编制出版《药品红外光谱集》作为国家标准系列配套丛书，广泛用于药品的鉴别检验。1986年国家药典委员会组织中国药品生物制品检定所及湖北、北京、湖南、上海、天津、辽宁、黑龙江、江苏等省市药品检验所的部分专家组成编审组，负责绘制和审定图谱。1990年，出版了《药品红外光谱集》1990年版，该版光谱集共收载582幅图谱。为了适应光谱集编制工作的延续性，经编审组研究决定，分卷出版《药品红外光谱集》，1995年出版了第一卷，收载了光栅型红外分光光度计绘制的药品红外光谱图共685幅。2000年出版了第二卷，收载药品红外光谱图208幅，并全部改由傅立叶红外光谱仪绘制。2005年出版第三卷，共收载药品红外光谱图210幅（其中172个为新增品种，38个老品种重新绘制了图谱）。2010年出版第四卷，共收载药品红外光谱图124幅。2015年出版第五卷，共收载药品红外光谱图94幅。凡在《中华人民共和国药典》和国家药品标准中收载红外鉴别或检查的品种，除特殊情况外，本光谱集中均有相应收载，以供比对。《中华人民共和国药典》和国家药品标准中不另收载红外光谱图。其他光谱图可供药品检验中作对照用。

　　本光谱集所需的样品和资料得到了全国各省、市、自治区药品检验所及有关单位的大力支持，在此一并致谢。对于本光谱集的不妥之处，希望各有关单位在实践过程中及时提出宝贵意见，以便予以修订。

国家药典委员会

2015 年 6 月

PREFACE

Infrared spectrophotometry is a means widely used to analyze organic compounds. As the high degree of specificity of the infrared spectrum for a given compound, infrared spectrophotometry is commonly adopted in pharmaceutical analysis combined with the other physical and chemical methods in the identification test of organic drug substances. With the number of organic drug substances increases continuously, especially their chemical structures are complicated or rare different in case of their analogs, the tests based on infrared spectrophotometry are always found to be an effective one when the usual methods for identification, such as color reactions, precipitation, crystal tests or Ultra-vis spectrophotometry, etc., are inadequate to differentiate the drug substances with closely related structures.

Identification tests of some drug substances based on infrared spectrophotometry were introduced for the first time into the Chinese Pharmacopoeia volume II , 1977 edition, and the infrared reference spectra were compiled in the appendix. In 1985, to meet the requirement of drug control in China, the Pharmacopoeia Commission entrusted some institutes for drug control to compile and publish the Atlas of Infrared Spectra of Drugs (1985) in which the infrared spectra for 423 drug substances supplied by domestic manufactures were recorded as the infrared reference spectra being adopted in specifications of pharmaceutical substances. Seeing that the infrared spectrophotometry had been adopted in the Chinese Pharmacopoeia as well as in other National Pharmaceutical Specifications and the number of specifications with tests based on infrared spectrophotometry was increasing steadily, there was a demand for further extension of this work. So the Atlas was officially published as a companion volume of National Pharmaceutical Specifications. Therefore, the Commission organized a collaborative study & reviewing experts group, composed of scientists from National Institute for the Control of Pharmaceutical and Biological Products, Hubei, Beijing, Hunan, Shanghai, Tianjin, Liaoning, Jiangsu and Heilongjiang Institutes for Drug Control, to carry out the work of recording, examining, verifying and compiling the spectra. In 1990, the Atlas of Infrared Spectra of Drugs (1990 edition) including 582 infrared spectra of drug substances was published. For the sake of continuity of this work, the Atlas of Infrared Spectra of Drugs would be published volume by volume.

There were 685 infrared spectra of the drug substances recorded by Grating Infrared Spectrophotometer in the volume I published in 1995. The volume II published in 2000 included 208 infrared spectra of the drug substances, which were all recorded by Fourier Transform Infrared Spectraphotometer instead. The volume III published in 2005 included 210 infrared spectra of the drug substances (172 new spectra and 38 re-recorded ones). The volume IV published in 2010 consists

of 124 infrared spectra of the drug substances. The volume V published in 2015 consists of 94 infrared spectra of the drug substances. With the exception of particular situations, the corresponding spectra in this Atlas are used as reference spectra of drug substances for identification or purity test required in monographs concerned in the Chinese Pharmacopoeia as well as in other National Pharmaceutical Specifications, which will not include infrared spectrum any more. The other spectra in this Atlas may be used also as reference spectra in pharmaceutical analysis.

In the course of compilation, the group is indebted to the full support in providing the specimens of drug substances and reference materials from various Institutes for Drug Control as well as manufacturers throughout the country.

All comments and suggestions concerning the contents of the Atlas will be welcome and subjected to careful consideration and necessary amendments be made for inclusion in subsequent supplement or next volume.

Pharmacopoeia Commission of P.R. China

说　　　　明

一、《药品红外光谱集》每卷有三个部分，即说明、光谱图和索引。光谱图系由《中华人民共和国药典》、国家药品标准中所收载的药品，用红外光谱仪录制而得。每幅光谱图并记载该药品的中文名、英文名、结构式、分子式、光谱号及试样的制备方法等。

索引有中文名索引、英文名索引、分子式索引，索引中列出的数字系指光谱号。

二、红外光谱仪

本光谱集第五卷所收载的光谱图系由不同型号的傅立叶红外光谱仪录制，再用伯乐 WIN-IR 软件统一格式化。

三、光谱图的录制

除少数为鉴别药品必需的有关化合物外，本光谱集所收载的药品，均符合其药品质量标准的规定。

试样的制备

1. 压片法　取供试品约 1mg，置玛瑙研钵中，加入干燥的溴化钾或氯化钾细粉约 200mg，充分研磨混匀，移置于直径为 13mm 的压模中，使铺布均匀，抽真空约 2min 后，加压至 0.8 ～ 1 GPa，保持 2 ～ 5min，除去真空，取出制成的供试片，目视检查应均匀透明，无明显颗粒（也可采用其他直径的压模制片，样品与分散剂的用量可相应调整以制得浓度合适的片子）。将供试片置于仪器的样品光路中，并扣除用同法制成的空白溴化钾或氯化钾片的背景，录制光谱图。

对溴化钾或氯化钾的质量要求　用溴化钾或氯化钾制成空白片，录制光谱图，基线应大于 75% 透光率；除在 3440cm^{-1} 及 1630cm^{-1} 附近因残留或附着水而呈现一定的吸收峰外，其他区域不应出现大于基线 3% 透光率的吸收谱带。

2. 糊法　取供试品约 5mg，置玛瑙研钵中，滴加少量液状石蜡或其他适宜的液体，制成均匀的糊状物，取适量夹于两个溴化钾片（每片重约 150mg）之间，作为供试片；以溴化钾约 300mg 制成空白片作为背景补偿，录制光谱图。亦可用其他适宜的盐片夹持糊状物。

3. 膜法　参照上述糊法所述的方法，将液体供试品铺展于溴化钾片或其他适宜的盐片中录制；或将供试品置于适宜的液体池内录制光谱图。若供试品为高分子聚合物，可先制成适宜厚度的薄膜，然后置样品光路中测定。

4. 溶液法　将供试品溶于适宜的溶剂内，制成 1% ～ 10% 浓度的溶液，置于 0.1 ～ 0.5 mm 厚度的液体池中录制光谱图，并以相同厚度装有同一溶剂的液体池作为背景补偿。

5. 衰减全反射法　将供试品均匀地铺展在衰减全反射棱镜的底面上，使紧密接触，依法录制反射光谱图。

6. 气体法　采用光路长度约为 10cm 的气体池，首先将气体池抽真空，然后充以适当压力（例如 30 ～ 50mmHg) 的供试气体，录制光谱图。

制图

本卷中光谱图的横坐标为波数（cm^{-1}），纵坐标为透光率（$T\%$）。

本卷收载的光谱图，系用分辨率为 $2cm^{-1}$ 条件绘制，基线一般控制在 90% 透光率以上，供试品取量一般控制在使其最强吸收峰在 10% 透光率以下。

四、光谱图的使用

1. 凡《中华人民共和国药典》、国家药品标准已收载用红外光谱法作为鉴别的原料药，本卷中收载的相应光谱图供比对用。

2. 本卷光谱图的波数范围为 4000 ～ $400cm^{-1}$，但有的红外光谱仪的光谱录制范围不同，用此类仪器录制的光谱图，除另有规定外，亦可使用本光谱集所收载的光谱图中相应的波数区间比对。所用仪器的性能应符合《中华人民共和国药典》通则 0402 红外分光光度法项下的要求。

3. 固体药品在测定时，可能由于晶型的影响，致使录制的光谱图与本光谱集所收载的光谱图不一致，遇此情况，应按本光谱集中各相应光谱图中备注的方法或该品种正文中规定的方法进行预处理后，再行录制。

4. 采用压片法时，影响图谱形状的因素较多，使用本光谱集对照时，应注意供试片的制备条件对图谱形状及各谱带的相对吸收强度可能产生的影响。

压片时，若样品（盐酸盐）与溴化钾之间不发生离子交换反应，则采用溴化钾作为制片基质。否则，盐酸盐样品制片时必须使用氯化钾基质。

5. 常用的傅立叶变换红外光谱仪系单光束型仪器。因此，应注意二氧化碳和水汽等的大气干扰，必要时，应采取适当措施（如采用干燥氮气吹扫）予以改善。

6. 为便于光谱的比对，本光谱集收载了聚苯乙烯薄膜的光谱图。在比对所测药品的光谱图与本光谱集所收载的药品的光谱图时，宜首先在测定药品所用的仪器上录制聚苯乙烯薄膜的光谱图，与本光谱集收载的聚苯乙烯薄膜的光谱图加以比较，由于仪器间的分辨率存在差异及不同操作条件的影响，聚苯乙烯薄膜光谱图的比较，将有助于药品光谱图比对时的判断。

7. 由于图谱的质量或供试品的多晶型等原因，有些化合物的光谱图作了重新绘制，并收入后续卷中。若同一化合物的光谱图在不同卷中均有收载，用于鉴别时以后卷光谱图作为比对依据，前卷光谱图仅作为参考。

NOTICES

I . Each volume, the Atlas of Infrared Spectra of Drugs, consists of three parts: notices, spectra and indexes. The spectra were recorded using an infrared spectrophotometer from the drug substances described in the Chinese Pharmacopoeia and National Pharmaceutical Specifications promulgated by China Food and Drug Administration. Under each spectrum are described both Chinese and English generic names, structural and molecular formulas, spectrum number and preparation method for sample of the drug substance concerned.

Indexes are arranged in Chinese titles, English titles as well as molecular formulas of the drug substances, respectively. The numeral listed in the index indicates the spectrum number.

II . Infrared spectrophotometer

The spectra in Volume V were recorded using various models of Fourier Transform Infrared Spectrophotometers and all these digital raw IR data from various FTIRs were processed with Bio-Rad WIN-IR software to achieve the format unification of spectra.

III . Recording of spectra

In Volume IV , all drug substances used for recording the spectra comply with their requirements described in the monographs concerned with the exception of a few related compounds which are necessary in identification test of certain drugs.

Procedures for preparation of samples

1. Disc Method

Triturate about 1mg of the substance being examined with approximate 200 mg of dried, finely powdered potassium bromide or potassium chloride in an agate mortar. Grind the mixture thoroughly and spread it uniformly in a die of 13 mm in diameter. Compress the mixture under vacuum with a pressure applied to the die of 0.8–1 GPa for 2 to 5 minutes, after the die assembly has been evacuated about 2 minutes. Remove the vacuum and take off the disc. The resultant disc should be uniform transparent and free from any obvious particles by visual inspection. When and if the die of other diameters is used, the dosages of sample and dispersive reagent should be adjusted accordingly to prepare the disc with suitable concentration. Mount the disc in a suitable holder and place it into the sample beam of the spectrophotometer. Place a similarly

prepared blank disc of potassium bromide or potassium chloride into the sample beam for background compensation. Record the spectrum with background deducted.

Quality Requirement for potassium bromide or potassium chloride Record the spectrum of a blank disc of potassium bromide or potassium chloride prepared as described above. The spectrum has a substantially flat baseline exhibiting no maxima with an absorbance greater than 3% of transmittance above the baseline, with the exception of maxima due to residual or absorbed water at about 3440 cm^{-1} and 1630 cm^{-1}. The baseline should be more than 75% of transmittance.

2. Mull method

Triturate about 5 mg of the substance being examined with a little amount of liquid paraffin or other suitable liquid to give a homogeneous creamy paste in an agate mortar. Compress and hold a portion of the mull between two flat potassium bromide plates (about 150 mg each). Record the spectrum by using a blank disc of potassium bromide with about 300 mg in weight for background compensation. Other suitable salt plates may be used instead of potassium bromide plates.

3. Film method

Use a capillary film of the liquid substance being examined held between two potassium bromide plates or other suitable salt plates with the method as described in the mull method. A filled cell of suitable thickness may be also used. For high polymer, prepare a film with suitable thickness. Mount the film in a suitable holder and place it into the sample beam. Record the spectrum.

4. Solution method

Prepare a solution of the substance being examined in a suitable solvent to the concentrations of 1%–10%. Place the solution in a filled cell with a thickness of 0.1 to 0.5 mm. Record the spectrum when a matched cell filled with the same solvent as background.

5. ATR method

Place the substance being examined in a manner of homogeneous and close contact with an ATR (Attenuated Total Reflectance) prism, and record its reflectance spectrum.

6. Gas method

Examine gases in a cell with optical path length of about 10cm. Evacuate the cell and fill the gas being examined to a suitable pressure (for example, 30–50mmHg). Record the spectrum.

Spectrum recording

The linear abscissa of the spectrum shows wave number (cm^{-1}) and the ordinate of the spectrum indicates transmittance (T%).

The spectra were recorded at 2 cm^{-1} resolution. In general, the baseline in spectrum was controlled to be more than 90% transmittance and the transmittance of the

strongest absorbance peak was controlled to be less than 10% by appropriately adjusting the quantity of substance being examined.

Ⅳ. Uses of the spectra

1. The corresponding spectra in this Atlas are used as reference spectra for drug substance when the identification by the use of infrared spectrophotometry is required in monographs of the Chinese Pharmacopoeia and National Pharmaceutical Specifications promulgated by China Food and Drug Administration.

2. In volume Ⅳ, the spectrum was scanned in the range from $4000cm^{-1}$ to $400cm^{-1}$. However, the spectrum recorded on different models of infrared spectrophotometer, which may have different scanning range, can be compared with the relevant spectrum included in this volume within the corresponding spectrum region. Of course, the performance of the instrument used should meet the requirements of *Infrared Spectrophotometry* as described in the appendix 0402 of the Chinese Pharmacopoeia.

3. Due to polymorphism, the difference between the spectrum recorded from the substance being examined and the relevant spectrum included in this volume may occur. In this case, the preparation method of the substance being examined as described in the note of the spectrum or that described in the monograph should be followed.

4. Various factors may affect the character of spectrum recorded by disc method. Therefore, the possible influence of preparation conditions of disc to the positions and the relative intensities of the absorbance bands should be considered when the spectrum in this volume is used for comparison.

If no ion-exchange reaction happens between the substance (chloride salts) being examined and the matrix when preparing disc, potassium bromide should be used as matrix for all solid specimens. Otherwise, potassium chloride must be used as matrix for chloride salts.

5. Care should be taken to the interference of atmosphere including carbon dioxide and water, because FT–IR spectrophotometer is usually a single beam type instrument. Some suitable measures, such as blow with dried nitrogen, should be adopted if necessary.

6. A spectrum of a polystyrene film is included in this volume for the convenience of comparison. It is suggested that a polystyrene spectrum is recorded on the instrument being used for examination of the substance being examined. Both spectra should be compared at first to observe any possible differences due to the potential variations of resolving power and operating conditions of the instruments being used. With reference to these factors, it would be useful for assessing the concordance of the spectrum of the substance being examined with that of the reference spectrum in this volume.

7. Due to some reasons, such as the quality of spectrum or polymorphism of the substance being examined, the spectra of some compounds were rerecorded and inscrolled in the subsequent volume. If the spectra of some compounds were inscrolled in different volumes, the spectrum inscrolled in latter volume should be used as criteria for identification, and the spectrum in former volume only as reference.

聚苯乙烯薄膜标准红外光谱图

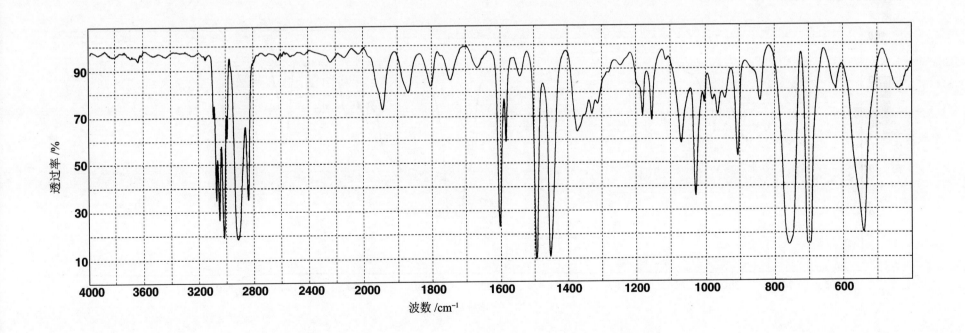

波数 /cm⁻¹

中文名：消旋羟蛋氨酸钙

英文名：D,L-α-Hydroxymethionine Calcium

分子式：$C_{10}H_{18}CaO_6S_2$

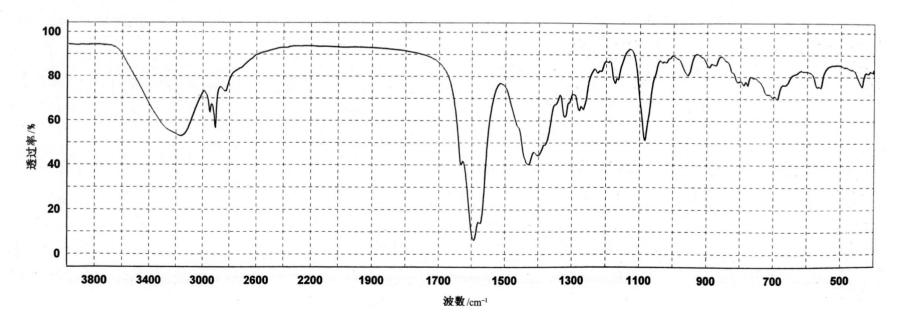

试样制备：KBr 压片法

备注：在 60℃减压干燥 4 小时后测定。

Note: Dry at 60℃ in vacuum for 4 hours.

光谱号　1229

中文名：胆酸

英文名：Cholic Acid

分子式：C_{24}H_{40}O_5

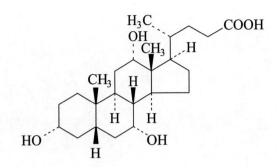

试样制备：KBr 压片法

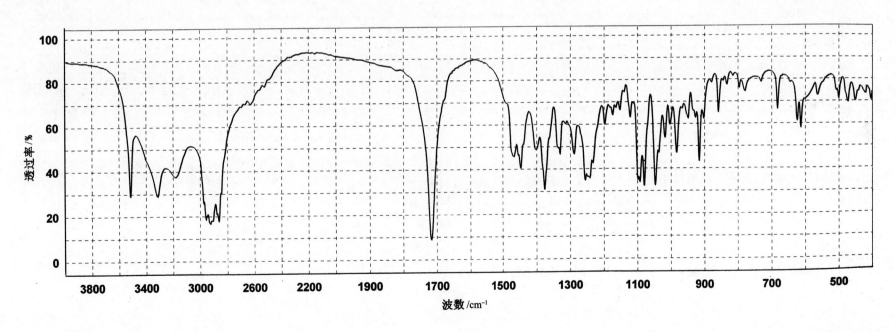

中文名：地塞米松棕榈酸酯

英文名：Dexamethasone Palmitate

分子式：C$_{38}$H$_{59}$FO$_6$

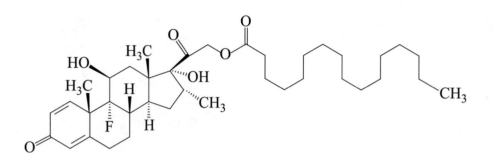

试样制备：KBr 压片法

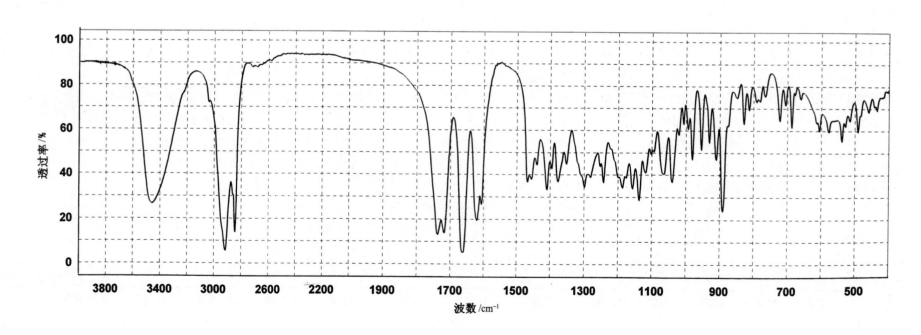

光谱号 1231

中文名：地西他滨

英文名：Decitabine

分子式：C₈H₁₂N₄O₄

试样制备：KBr 压片法

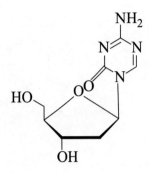

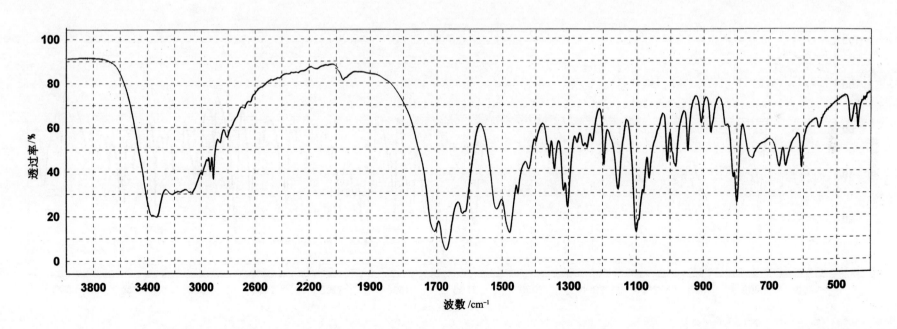

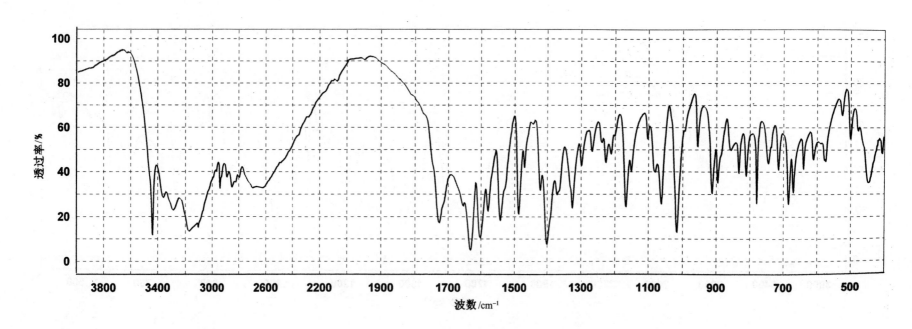

中文名：恩替卡韦

英文名：Entecavir

分子式：C₁₂H₁₅N₅O₃

试样制备：KBr 压片法

光谱号　1233

中文名：二氮嗪

英文名：Diazoxide

分子式：C$_8$H$_7$ClN$_2$O$_2$S

试样制备：KBr 压片法

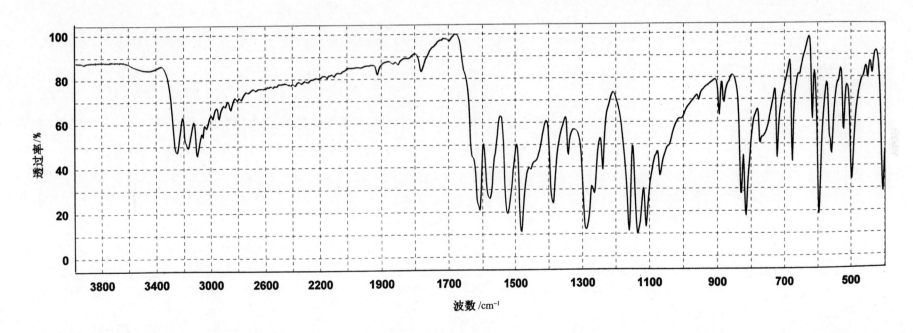

透过率/%

波数 /cm⁻¹

中文名：夫西地酸钠

英文名：Sodium Fusidate

分子式：C$_{31}$H$_{47}$NaO$_6$

试样制备：KBr 压片法

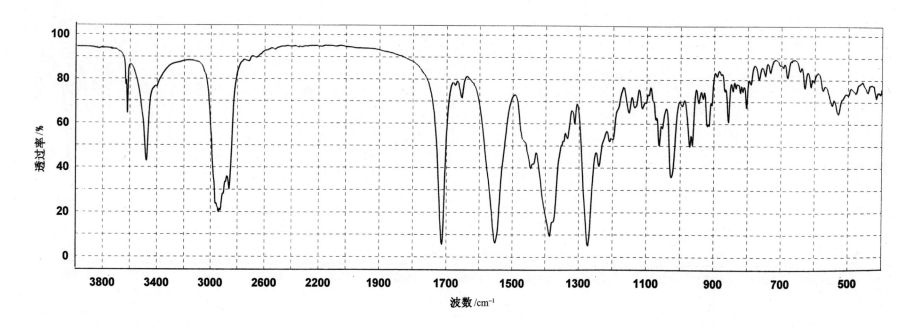

中文名: 富马酸阿奇霉素

英文名: Azithromycin Fumarate

分子式: $C_{38}H_{72}N_2O_{12} \cdot C_4H_4O_4$

试样制备: KBr 压片法

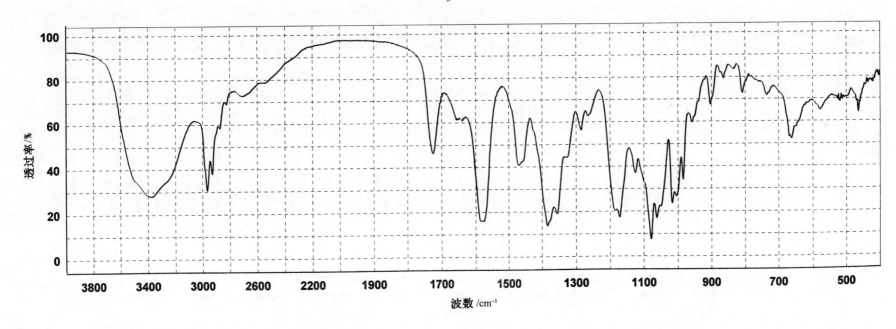

中文名：富马酸芦帕他定

英文名：Rupatadine Fumarate

分子式：$C_{26}H_{26}ClN_3 \cdot C_4H_4O_4$

试样制备：KBr 压片法

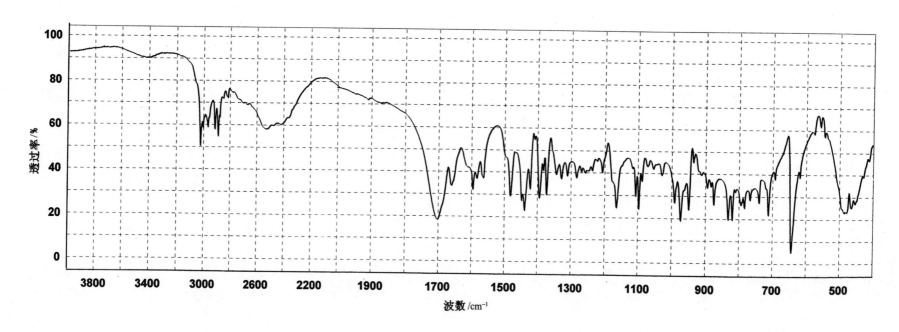

光谱号　1237

中文名：甘露醇

英文名：Mannitol

分子式：C₆H₁₄O₆

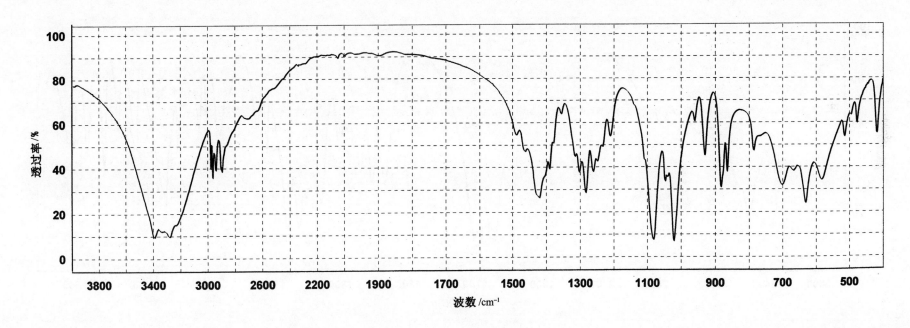

试样制备：KBr 压片法

光谱号 1238

中文名：枸橼酸

英文名：Citric Acid

分子式：$C_6H_8O_7 \cdot H_2O$

试样制备：KBr 压片法

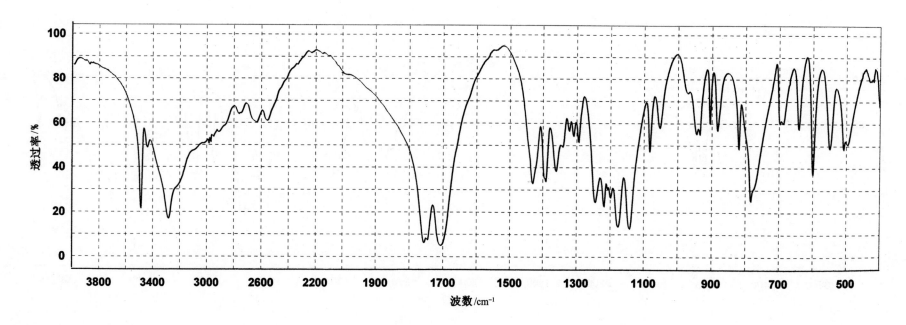

光谱号　1239

中文名：吗多明

英文名：Molsidomine

分子式：$C_9H_{14}N_4O_4$

试样制备：KBr 压片法

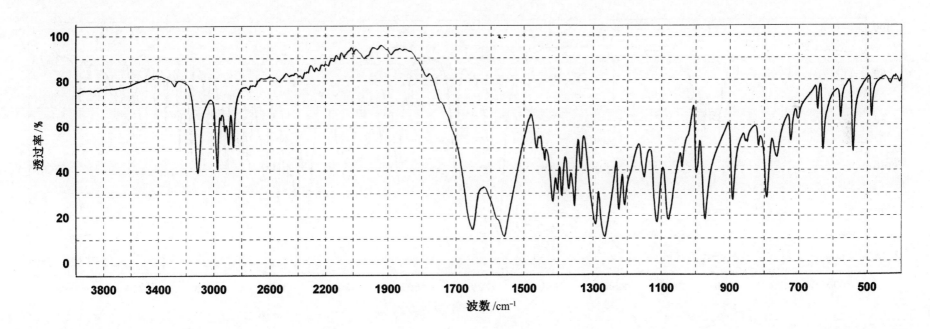

中文名：吗替麦考酚酯

英文名：Mycophenolate Mofetil

分子式：C$_{23}$H$_{31}$NO$_7$

试样制备：KBr 压片法

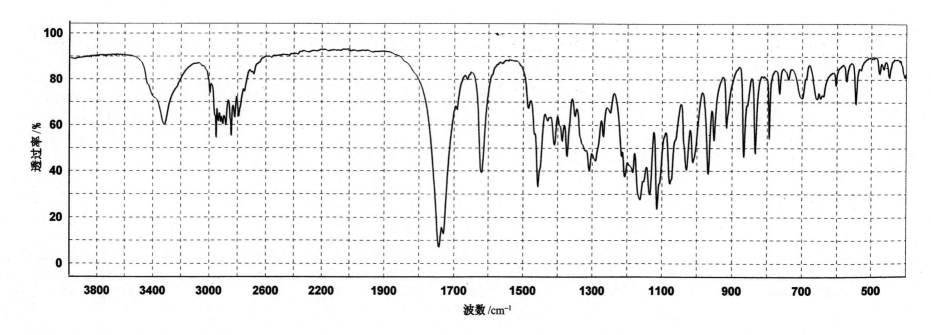

光谱号 1241

中文名：孟鲁司特钠

英文名：Montelukast Sodium

分子式：C_{35}H_{35}ClNNaO_3S

试样制备：KBr 压片法

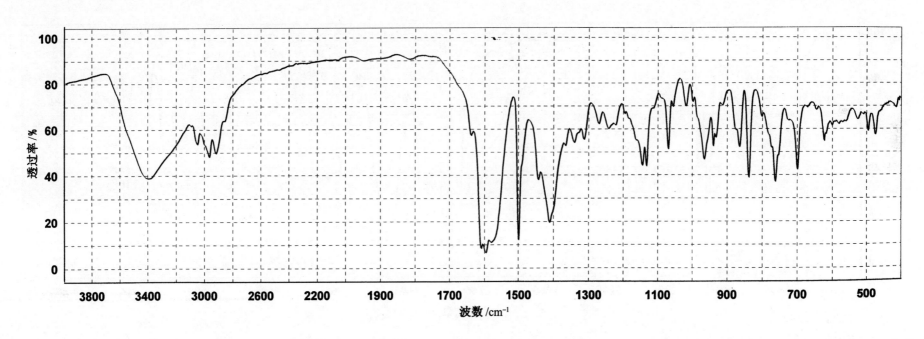

中文名：米格列奈钙

英文名：Mitiglinide Calcium

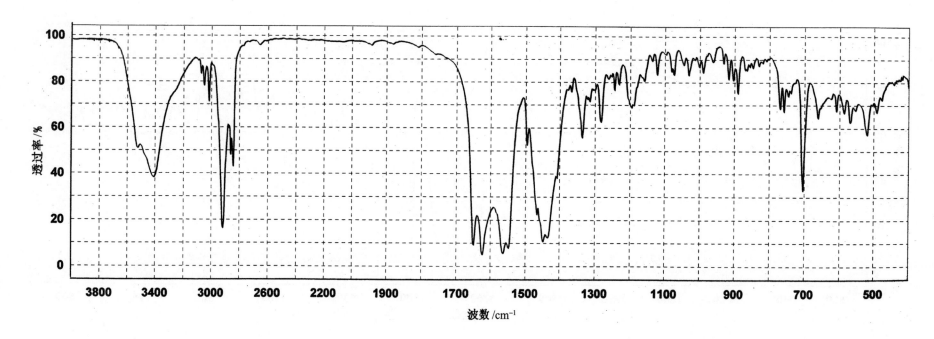

分子式：$C_{38}H_{48}CaN_2O_6 \cdot 2H_2O$

试样制备：KBr 压片法

光谱号　1243

中文名：罗舒伐他汀钙

英文名：Rosuvastatin Calcium

分子式：$C_{44}H_{54}F_2N_6O_{12}S_2Ca$

试样制备：KBr 压片法

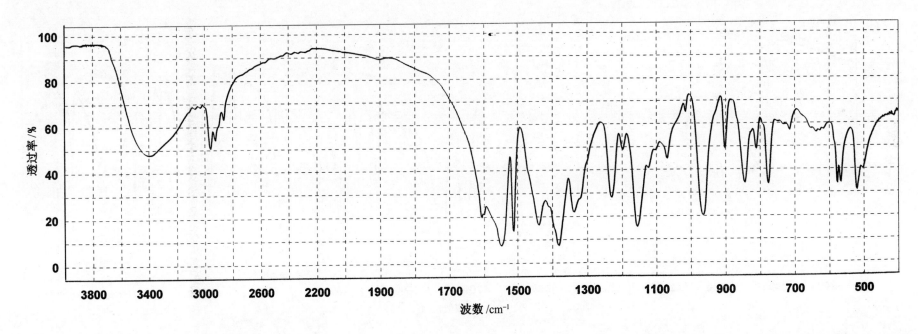

中文名：腺嘌呤

英文名：Adenine

分子式：C₅H₅N₅

试样制备：KBr 压片法

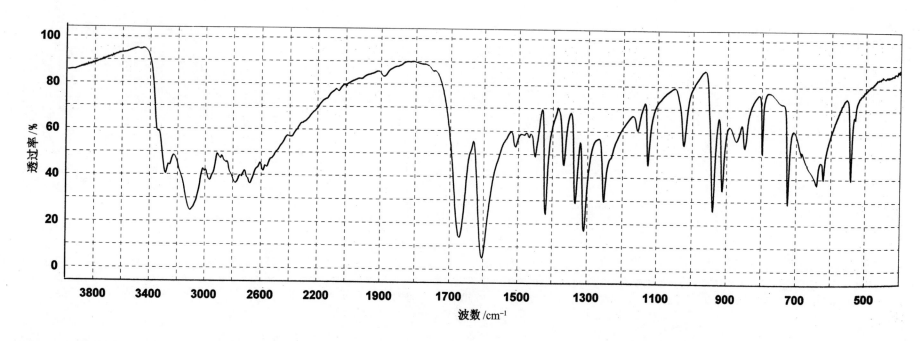

光谱号 1245

中文名：盐酸奥普力农

英文名：Olprinone Hydrochloride

分子式：C₁₄H₁₀N₄O・HCl・H₂O

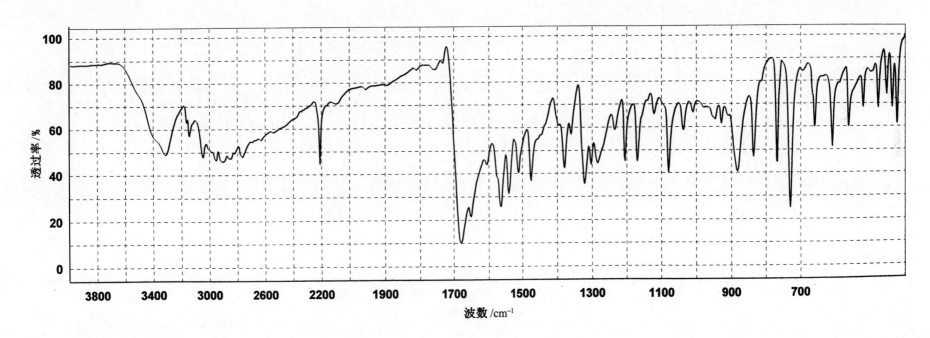

试样制备：KBr 压片法

光谱号　1246

中文名：盐酸甲砜霉素甘氨酸酯

英文名：Thiamphenicol Glycinate Hydrochloride

分子式：$C_{14}H_{18}Cl_2N_2O_6S \cdot HCl$

试样制备：KBr 压片法

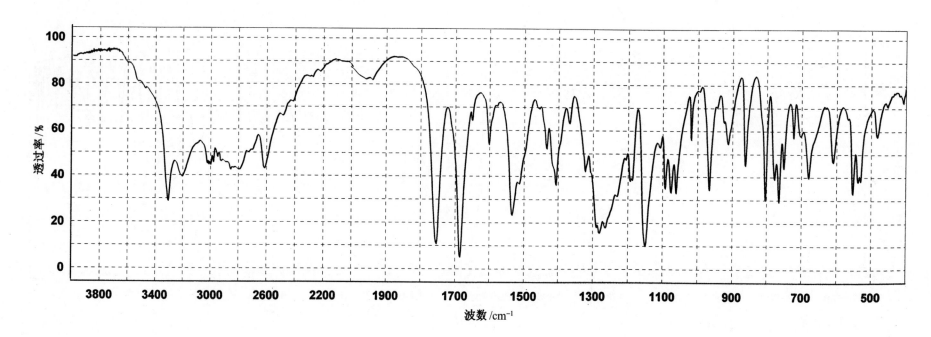

光谱号　1247

中文名：盐酸罗沙替丁醋酸酯

英文名：Roxatidine Acetate Hydrochloride

分子式：C₁₉H₂₈N₂O₄·HCl

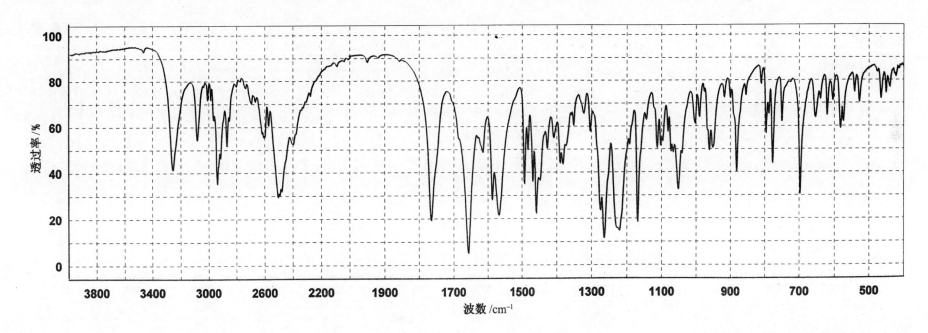

试样制备：KBr 压片法

光谱号 1248

中文名：依帕司他

英文名：Epalrestat

分子式：C₁₅H₁₃NO₃S₂

试样制备：KBr 压片法

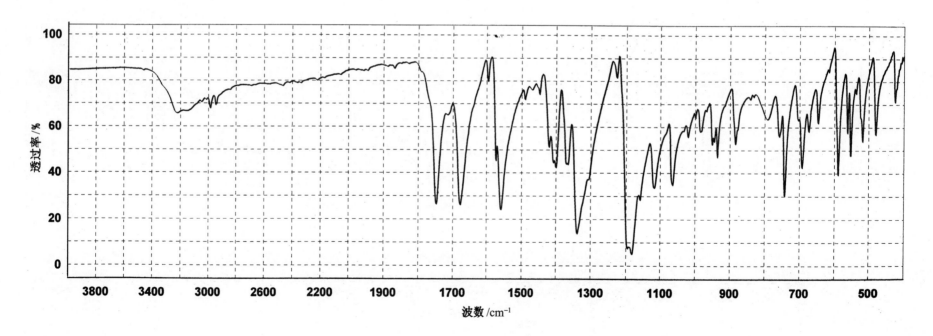

光谱号　1249

中文名：利福布汀

英文名：Rifabutin

分子式：C₄₆H₆₂N₄O₁₁

试样制备：KBr 压片法

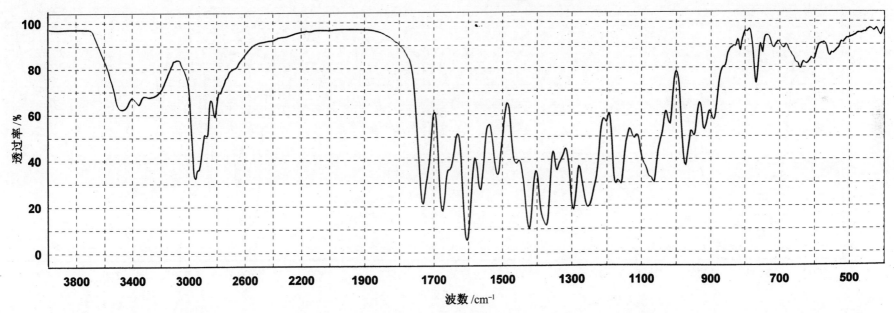

透过率 /%

波数 /cm⁻¹

中文名：磷霉素钠

英文名：Fosfomycin Sodium

分子式：C₃H₅Na₂O₄P

试样制备：KBr 压片法

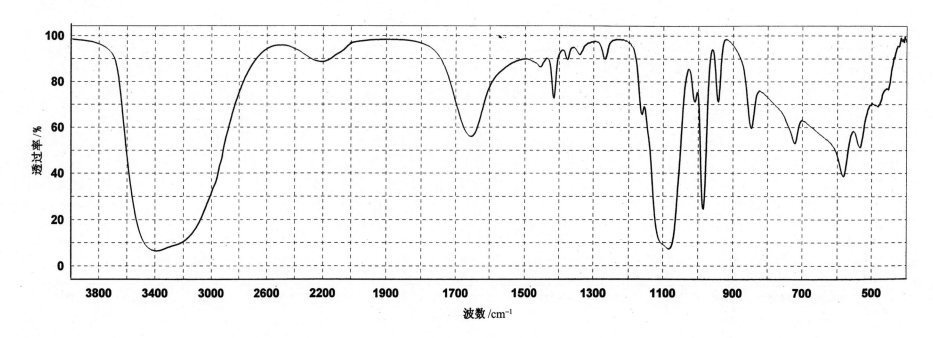

光谱号　1251

中文名：丙戊酸半钠

英文名：Valproate Semisodium

分子式：(C₁₆H₃₁NaO₄)ₙ

试样制备：KBr 压片法

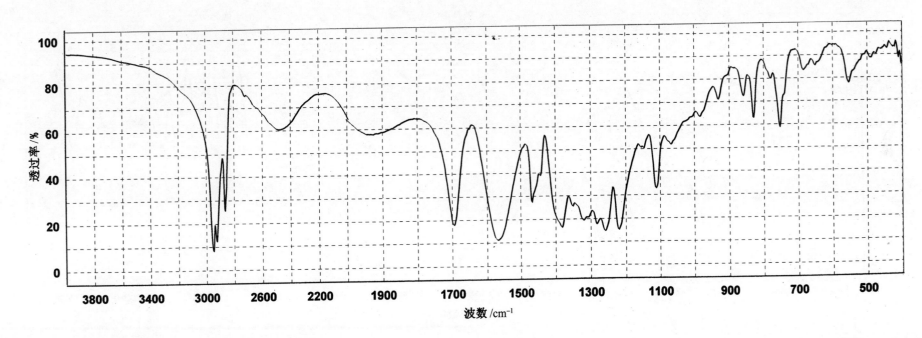

中文名：西司他丁钠

英文名：Cilastatin Sodium

分子式：C$_{16}$H$_{25}$N$_2$NaO$_5$S

试样制备：KBr 压片法

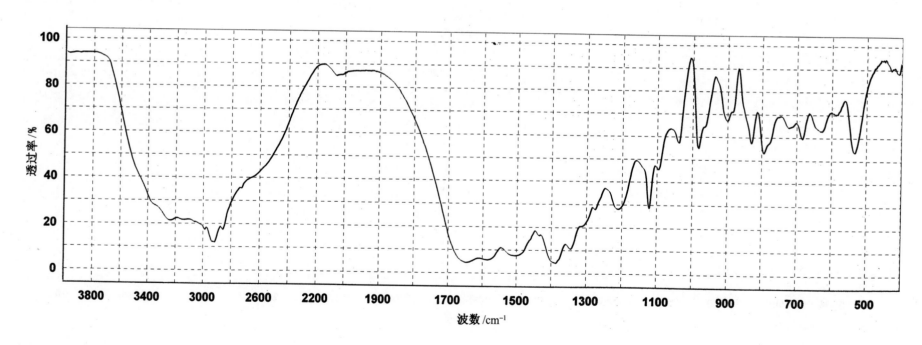

光谱号 1253

中文名：亚胺培南

英文名：Imipenem

分子式：$C_{12}H_{17}N_3O_4S \cdot H_2O$

试样制备：KBr 压片法

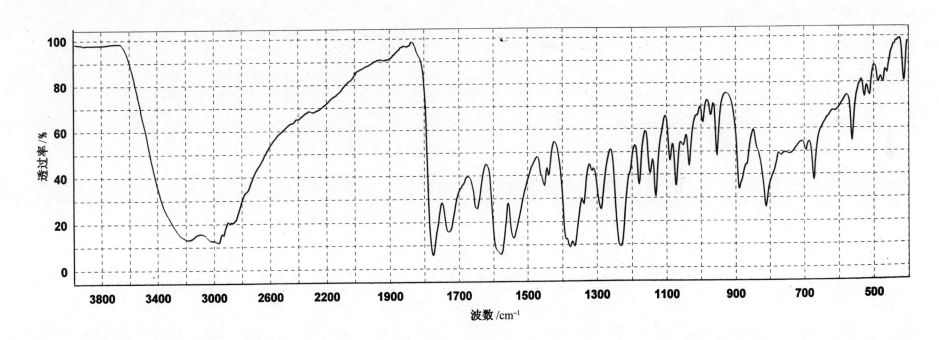

中文名：盐酸氮芥

英文名：Chlormethine Hydrochloride

分子式：$C_5H_{11}Cl_2N \cdot HCl$

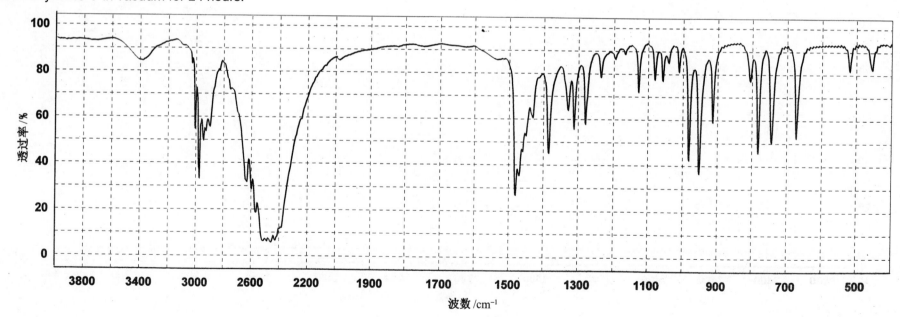

试样制备：KBr 压片法

备注：在 45℃减压干燥 24 小时后测定。

Note: Dry at 45℃ in vacuum for 24 hours.

光谱号 1255

中文名：盐酸多沙普仑

英文名：Doxapram Hydrochloride

分子式：C₂₄H₃₀N₂O₂·HCl·H₂O

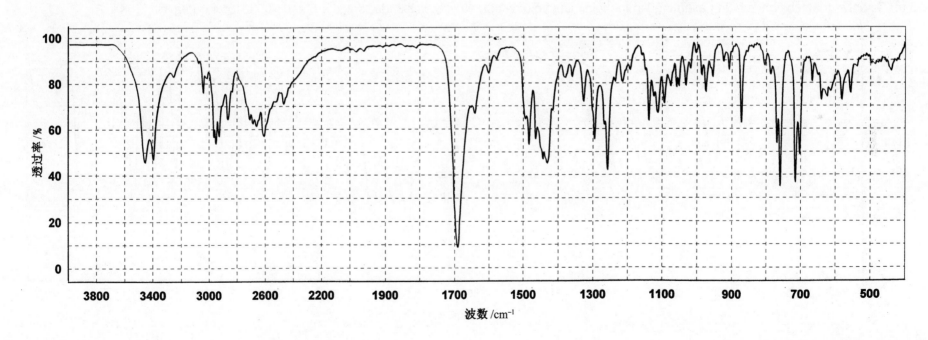

试样制备：KBr 压片法

中文名：盐酸洛哌丁胺

英文名：Loperamide Hydrochloride

分子式：C$_{29}$H$_{33}$ClN$_2$O$_2$·HCl

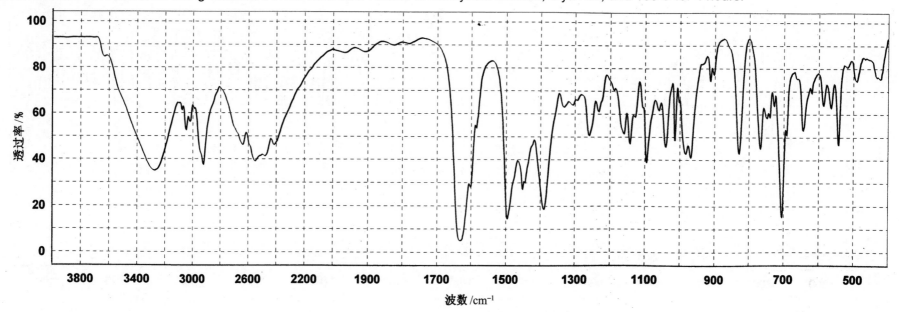

试样制备：KBr 压片法

备注：取样品适量，溶于二氯甲烷，挥干，105℃干燥4小时。

Note: Dissolve the substance being examined in the minimum volume of methylene chloride, dry in air, and 105℃ for 4 hours.

光谱号　1257

中文名：环吡酮胺

英文名：Ciclopirox Olamine

分子式：C₁₂H₁₇NO₂·C₂H₇NO

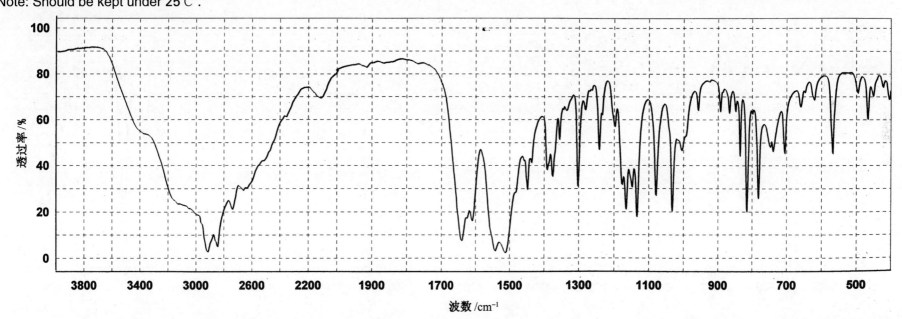

试样制备：糊法

备注：制备样品应在25℃以下保存。

Note: Should be kept under 25℃ .

中文名：磷酸川芎嗪

英文名：Ligustrazine Phosphate

分子式：C$_8$H$_{12}$N$_2$·H$_3$PO$_4$·H$_2$O

试样制备：KBr 压片法

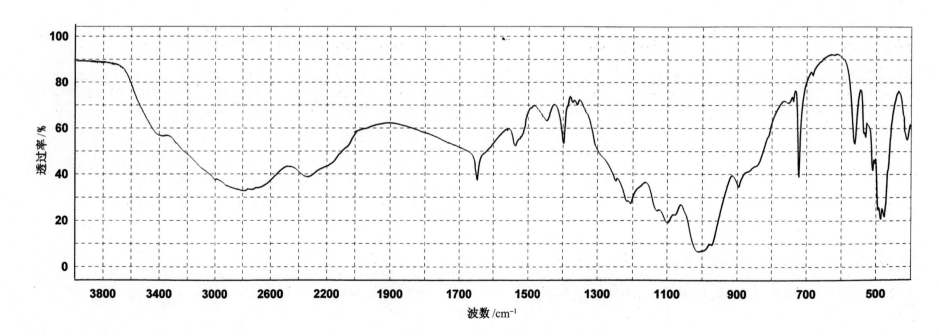

光谱号 1259

中文名：他唑巴坦

英文名：Tazobactam

分子式：C$_{10}$H$_{12}$N$_{4}$O$_{5}$S

试样制备：KBr 压片法

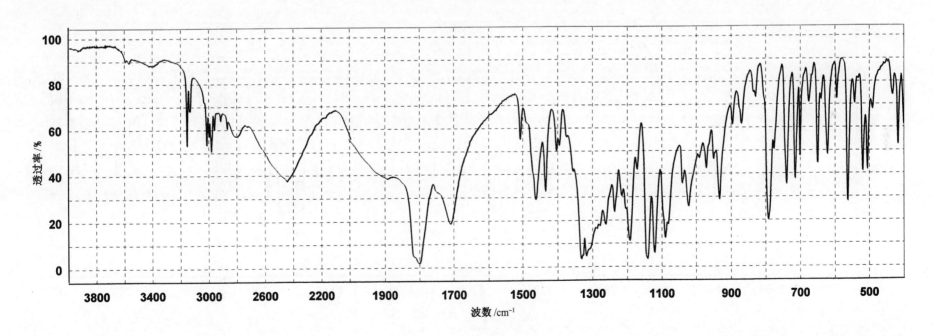

中文名：托西酸舒他西林

英文名：Sultamicillin Tosilate

分子式：$C_{25}H_{30}N_4O_9S_2 \cdot C_7H_8O_3S$

试样制备：糊法。
Preparation of sample: Mull method

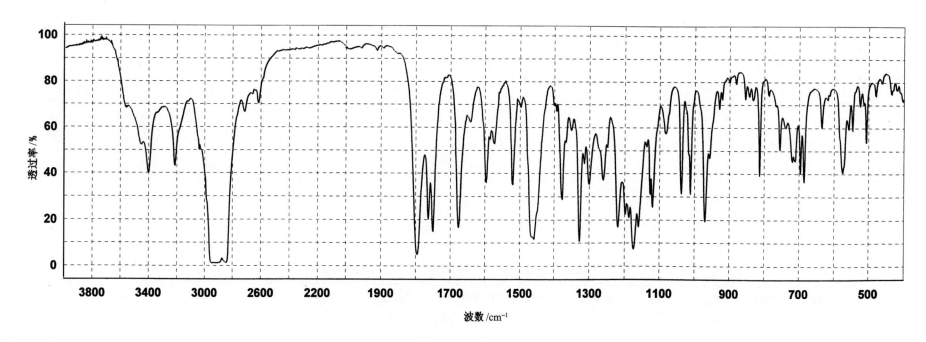

光谱号　1261

中文名：重酒石酸间羟胺

英文名：Metaraminol Bitartrate

分子式：C$_9$H$_{13}$NO$_2$ · C$_4$H$_6$O$_6$

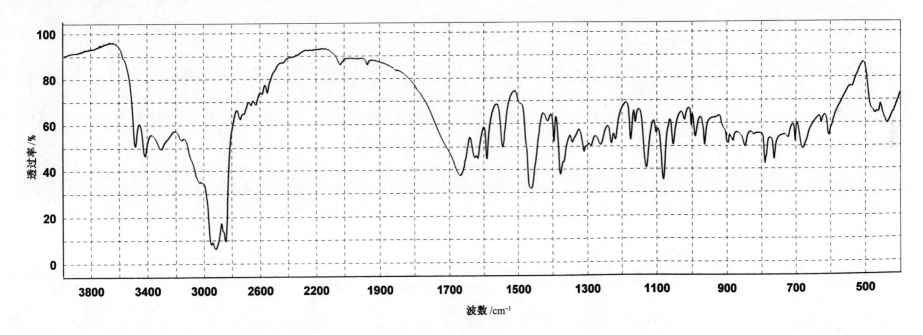

试样制备：糊法

Preparation of sample: Mull method.

中文名：谷氨酸

英文名：Glutamic Acid

分子式：C$_5$H$_9$NO$_4$

试样制备：KBr 压片法

备注：光谱号 958 图为 β 型谷氨酸，光谱号 1263 图为 α 型谷氨酸。

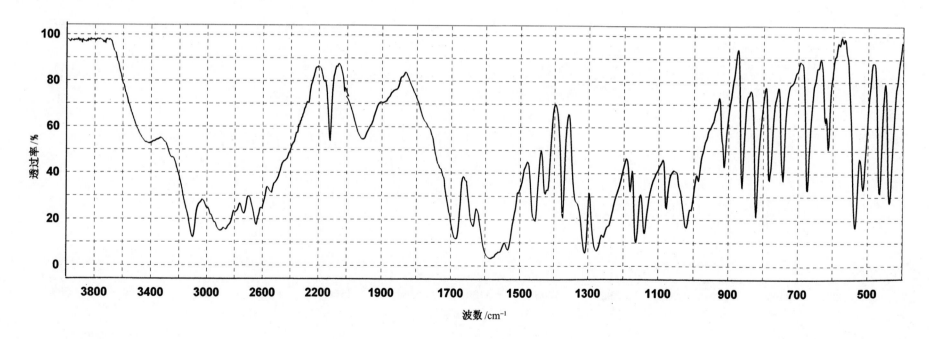

中文名：盐酸艾司洛尔

英文名：Esmolol Hydrochloride

分子式：C_{16}H_{25}NO_4·HCl

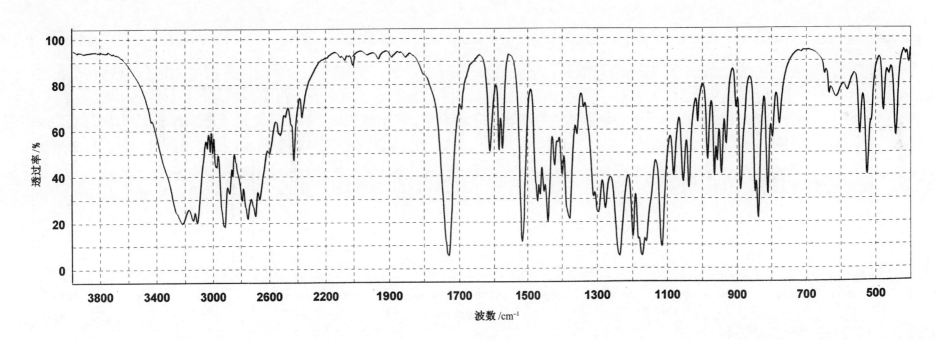

试样制备：KBr 压片法

中文名：盐酸文拉法辛

英文名：Venlafaxine Hydrochloride

分子式：$C_{17}H_{27}NO_2 \cdot HCl$

试样制备：KCl 压片法

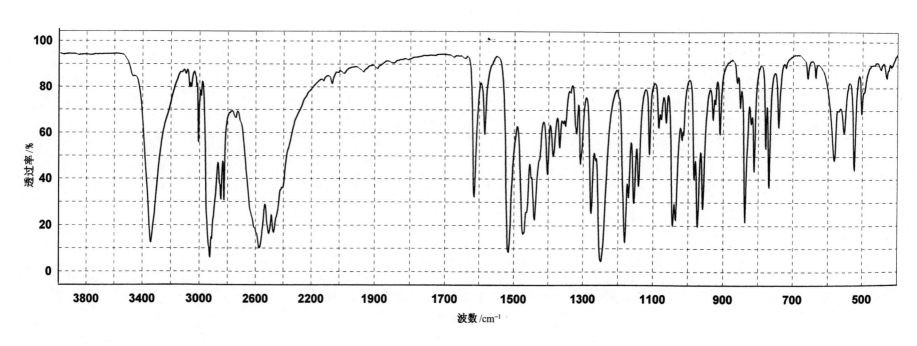

光谱号　1265

中文名：更昔洛韦

英文名：Ganciclovir

分子式：C$_9$H$_{13}$N$_5$O$_4$

试样制备：KBr 压片法

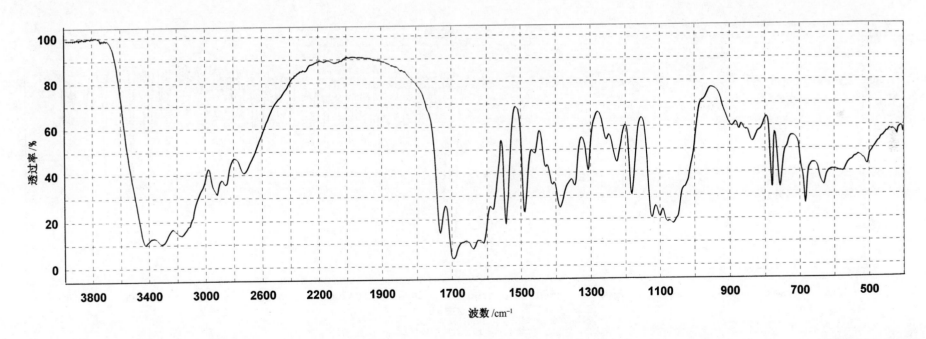

波数 /cm^{-1}

中文名：托吡卡胺

英文名：Tropicamide

分子式：C$_{17}$H$_{20}$N$_2$O$_2$

试样制备：KBr 压片法

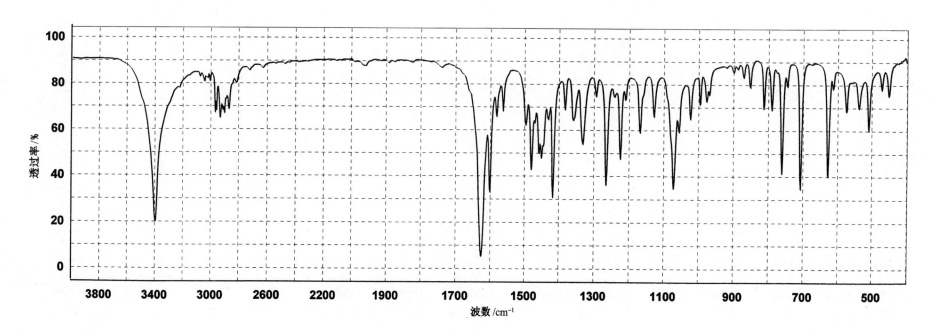

透过率 /%

波数 /cm⁻¹

光谱号　1267

中文名：甘油

英文名：Glycerol

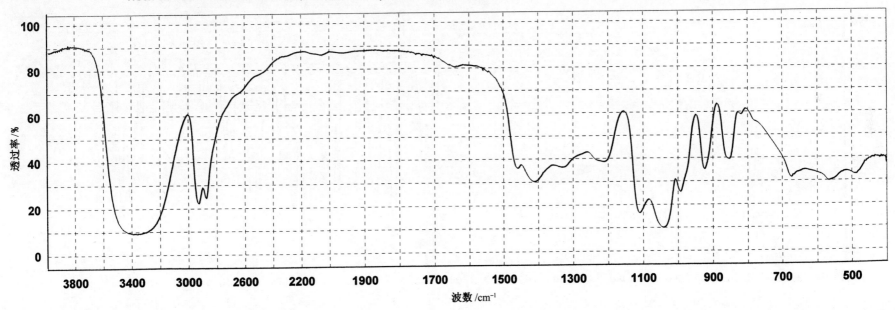

分子式：C$_3$H$_8$O$_3$

试样制备：取本品适量涂布于 KBr 空白片上，105℃加热 15 分钟后，立即测定。
Preparation of sample: Smear the substance being examined on a blank disc of potassium bromide, heat at 105℃ for 15 minutes, record the spectra immediately.

中文名：卡维地洛

英文名：Carvedilol

分子式：C_{24}H_{26}N_2O_4

试样制备：KBr 压片法

备注：取供试品 0.5g，置锥形瓶中，加异丙醇 5ml，水浴回流至完全溶解（约
10 分钟）。密塞静置，冷却，析出结晶，滤过，室温减压干燥后测定。

Note: To 0.5g in a conical flask add 5ml of 2-propanol and heat on a water-bath under a reflux condenser for about 10 minutes until dissolution is complete. Seal and allowed to stand without shaking .Cool. Crystals separate. Filter, and dry at room temperature in vacuum.

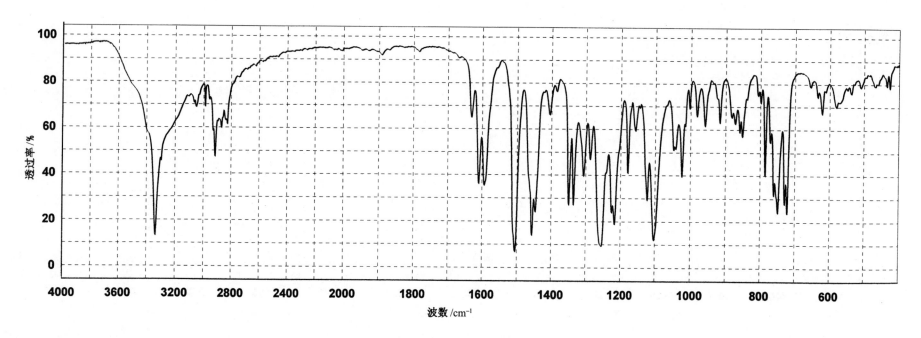

光谱号 1269

中文名：克霉唑

英文名：Clotrimazole

分子式：C$_{22}$H$_{17}$ClN$_2$

试样制备：KBr 压片法

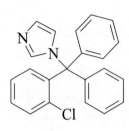

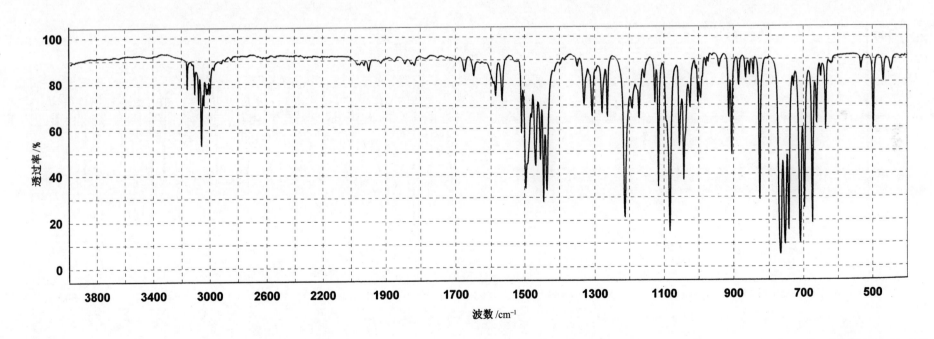

中文名：阿普唑仑

英文名：Alprazolam

分子式：C$_{17}$H$_{13}$ClN$_4$

试样制备：KBr 压片法

备注：取供试品适量，加少量无水乙醇，加热使溶解，置水浴上蒸干，105℃
干燥后测定。

Note: Dissolve a proper quantity in a little anhydrous ethanol with heat,
evaporate to dryness on water bath, dry at 105℃ .

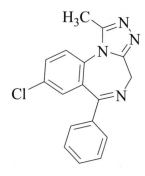

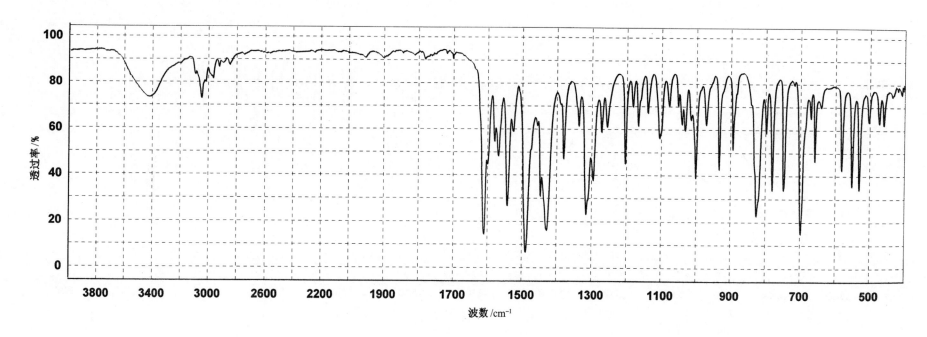

光谱号 1271

中文名：吡硫翁钠

英文名：Pyrithione Sodium

分子式：C_5H_4NNaOS

试样制备：KBr 压片法

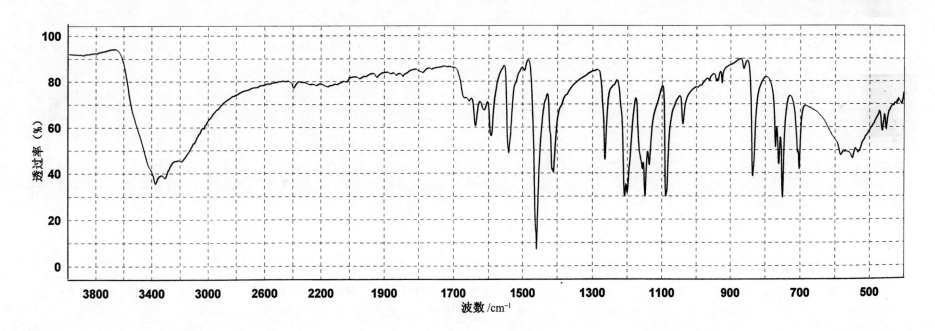

光谱号 1272

中文名：富马酸喹硫平

英文名：Quetiapine Fumarate

分子式：(C$_{21}$H$_{25}$N$_3$O$_2$S)$_2$·C$_4$H$_4$O$_4$

试样制备：KBr 压片法

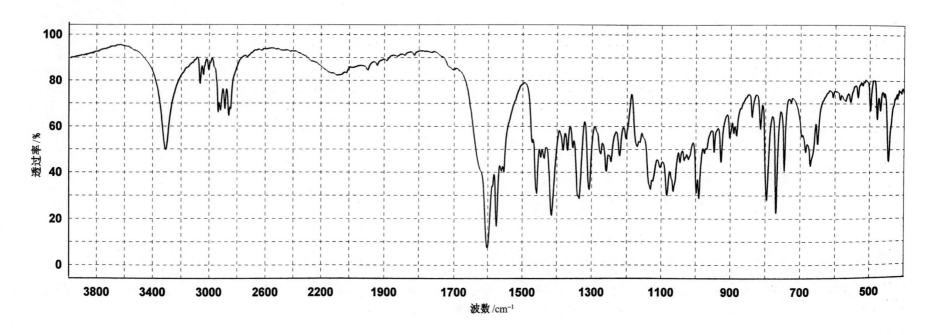

中文名：门冬酰胺

英文名：Asparagine

分子式：C₄H₈N₂O₃·H₂O

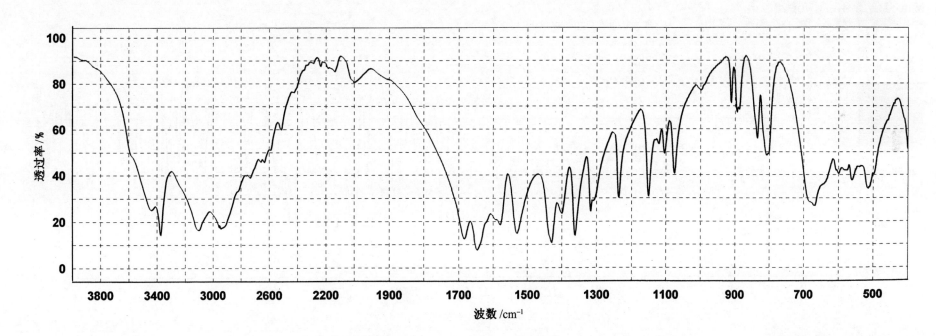

试样制备：KBr 压片法

中文名：吲达帕胺

英文名：Indapamide

分子式：C$_{16}$H$_{16}$ClN$_3$O$_3$S

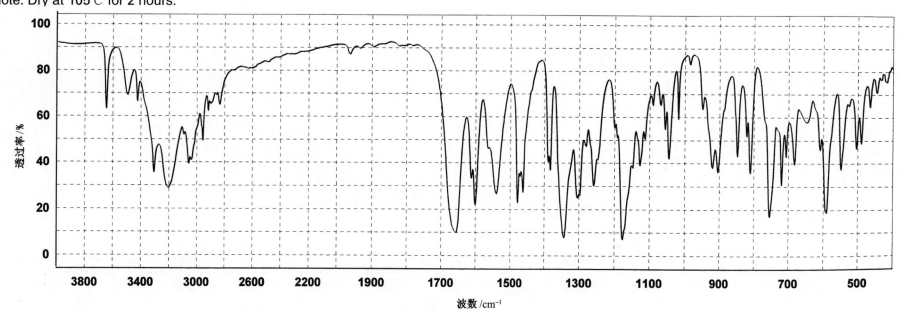

试样制备：KBr 压片法

备注：105℃干燥 2 小时后测定。

Note: Dry at 105℃ for 2 hours.

光谱号　1275

中文名：呱西替柳

英文名：Guacetisal

分子式：C$_{16}$H$_{14}$O$_5$

试样制备：KBr 压片法

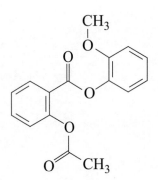

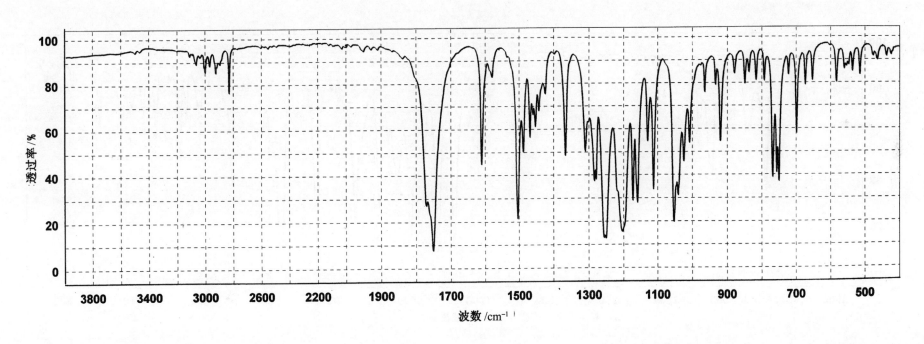

透过率 /%

波数 /cm^{-1}

光谱号　1276

中文名：曲昔派特

英文名：Troxipide

分子式：C$_{15}$H$_{22}$N$_2$O$_4$

试样制备：KBr 压片法

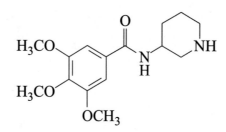

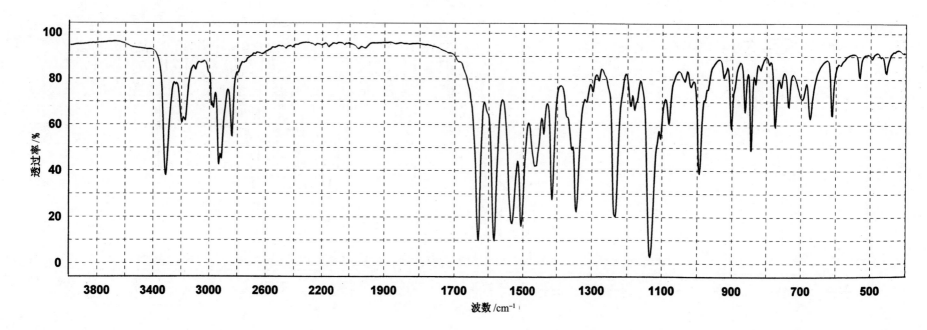

光谱号　1277

中文名：山梨醇

英文名：Sorbitol

分子式：C$_6$H$_{14}$O$_6$

试样制备：KBr 压片法

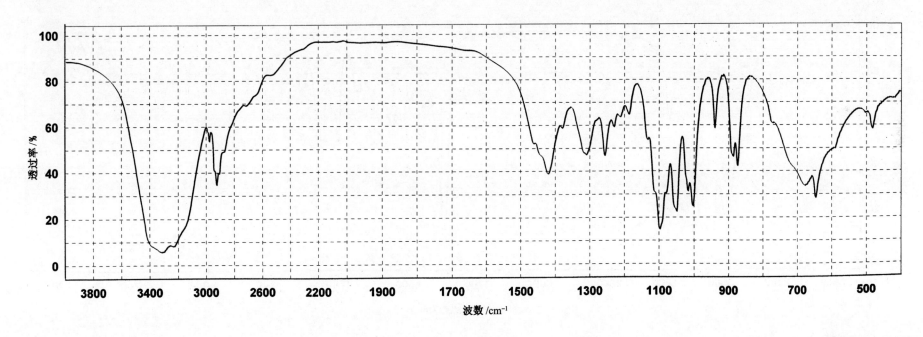

中文名：盐酸赛洛唑啉

英文名：Xylometazoline Hydrochloride

分子式：C$_{16}$H$_{24}$N$_2$·HCl

试样制备：KBr 压片法

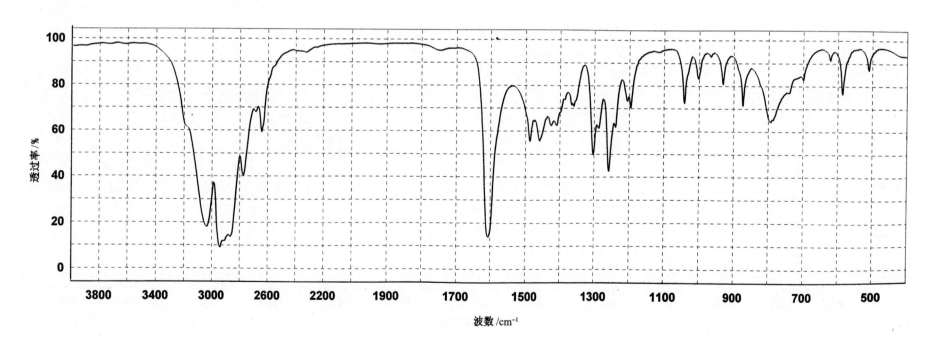

光谱号　1279

中文名：达卡巴嗪

英文名：Dacarbazine

分子式：$C_6H_{10}N_6O$

试样制备：KBr 压片法

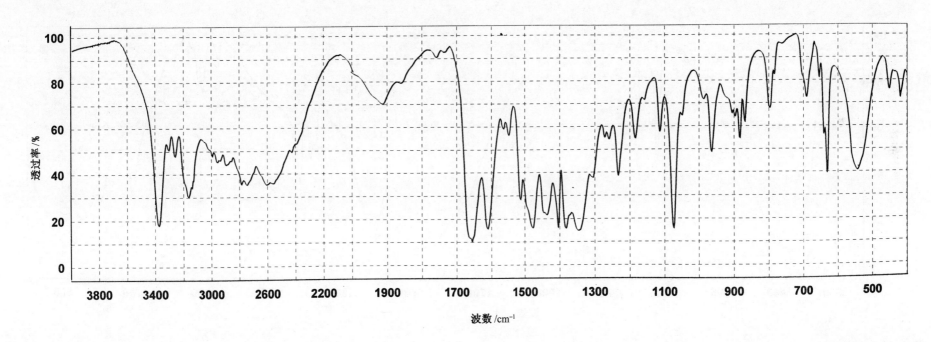

中文名：二巯丁二钠

英文名：Sodium Dimercaptosuccinate

分子式：C₄H₄Na₂O₄S₂·3H₂O

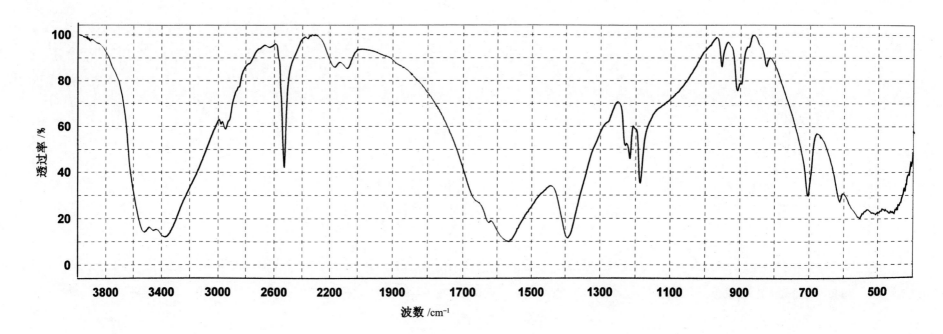

试样制备：KBr 压片法

光谱号　1281

中文名：盐酸舒托必利

英文名：Sultopride Hydrochloride

分子式：C$_{17}$H$_{26}$N$_2$O$_4$S · HCl

试样制备：KBr 压片法

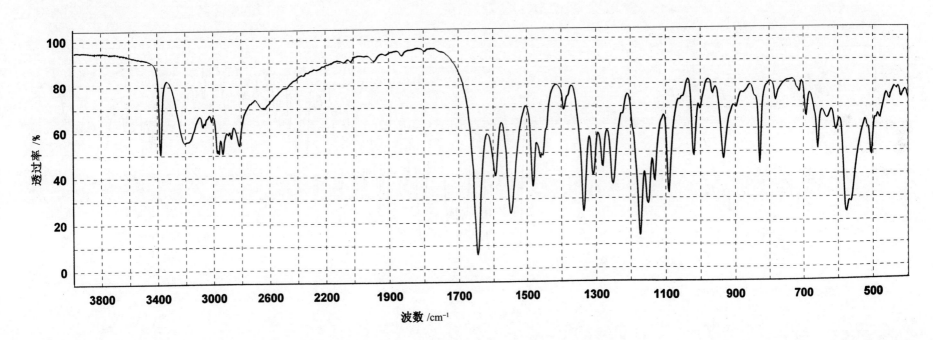

中文名：氨苄西林钠

英文名：Ampicillin Sodium

分子式：C$_{16}$H$_{18}$N$_3$NaO$_4$S

试样制备：KBr 压片法

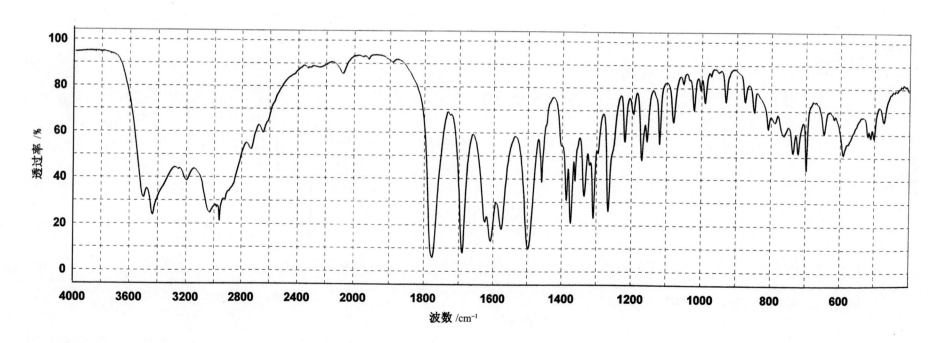

光谱号　1283

中文名：苄达赖氨酸

英文名：Bendazac Lysin

分子式：$C_6H_{14}N_2O_2 \cdot C_{16}H_{14}N_2O_3$

试样制备：KBr 压片法

备注：105℃干燥 1 小时后测定。

Note: Dry at 105℃ for 1 hour.

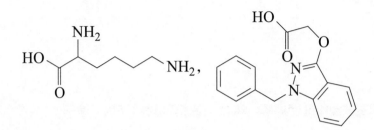

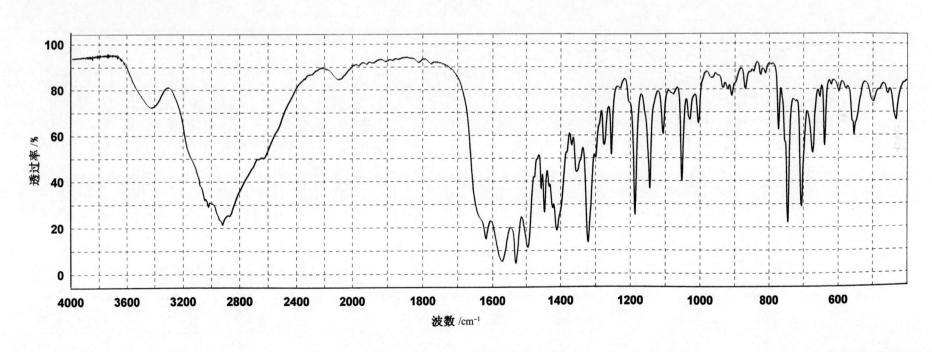

中文名：磷酸苯丙哌林

英文名：Benproperine Phosphate

分子式：C$_{21}$H$_{27}$NO·H$_3$PO$_4$

试样制备：膜法

备注：取本品约 20mg，加氨试液 1ml 使溶解，离心，取苯丙哌林（下层）涂于
溴化钾片上，测定。
Note: Dissolve about 20mg in 1ml of ammonia solution, centrifuge, smear
Benproperine (substrate) on a potassium bromide, record the spectra.

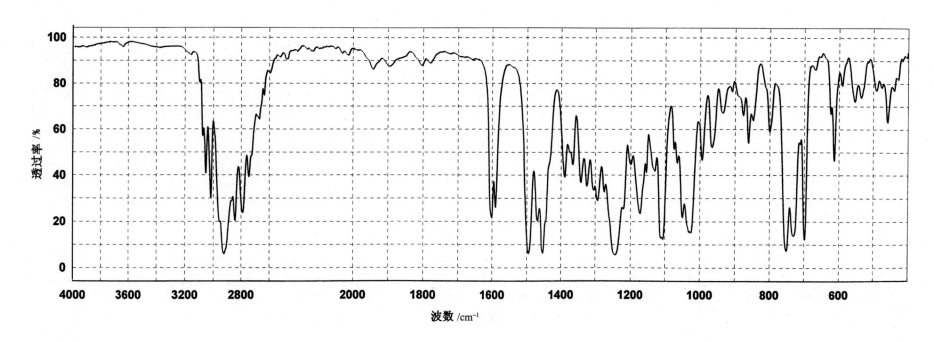

光谱号　1285

中文名：双羟萘酸奥克太尔

英文名：Oxantel Pamoate

分子式：C₁₃H₁₆N₂O・C₂₃H₁₆O₆

试样制备：KBr 压片法

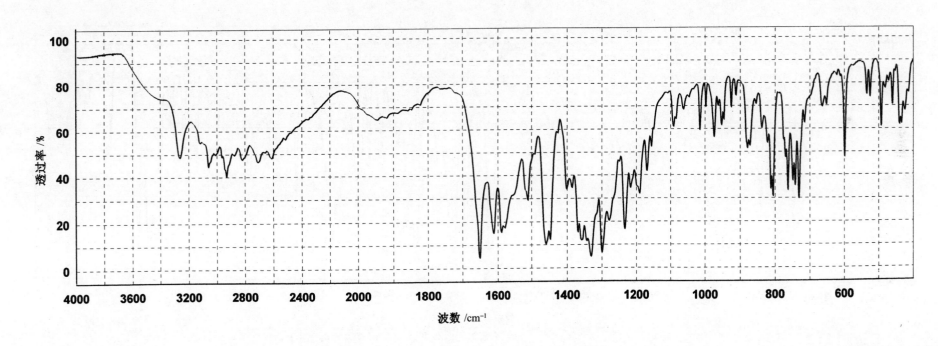

中文名：盐酸氯普鲁卡因

英文名：Chloroprocaine Hydrochloride

分子式：$C_{13}H_{19}ClN_2O_2 \cdot HCl$

试样制备：KBr 压片法

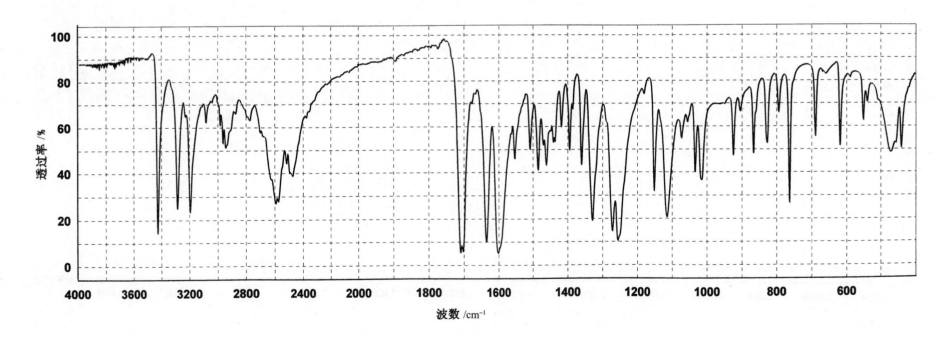

光谱号　1287

中文名：盐酸瑞芬太尼

英文名：Remifentanil Hydrochloride

分子式：C$_{20}$H$_{28}$N$_2$O$_5$・HCl

试样制备：KBr 压片

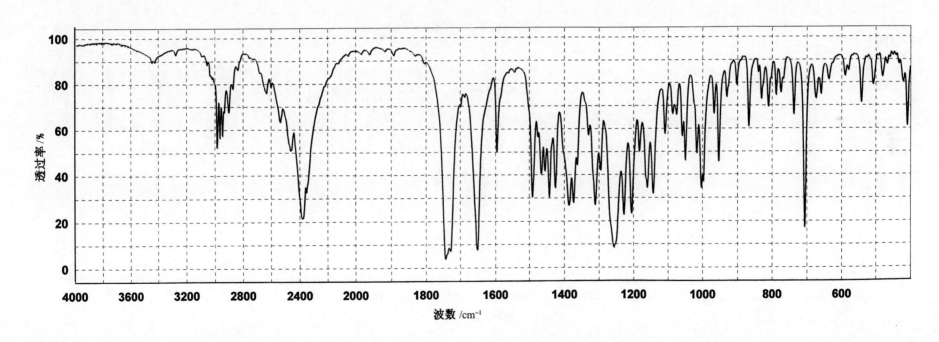

透过率 /%

波数 /cm^{-1}

中文名：咖啡因

英文名：Caffeine

分子式：C$_8$H$_{10}$N$_4$O$_2$

试样制备：KBr 压片法

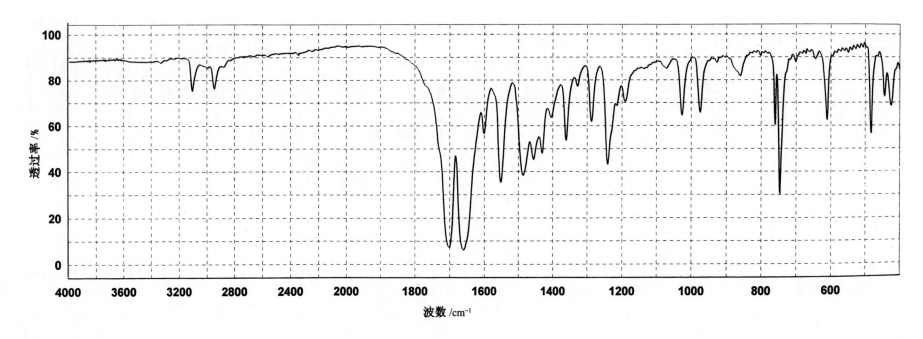

中文名：乙醇

英文名：Alcohol

分子式：C$_2$H$_6$O

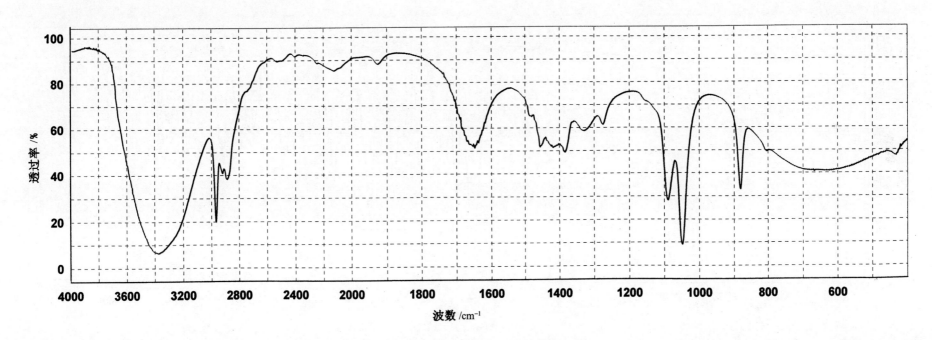

H$_3$C——OH

试样制备：液膜法
Preparation of sample: Liquid thin film

备注：使用自制的 KBr 片制液膜。
Note: Using a home-made potassium bromide.

透过率 /%

波数 /cm^{-1}

中文名：阿立哌唑

英文名：Aripiprazole

分子式：C$_{23}$H$_{27}$Cl$_2$N$_3$O$_2$

试样制备：KBr 压片法

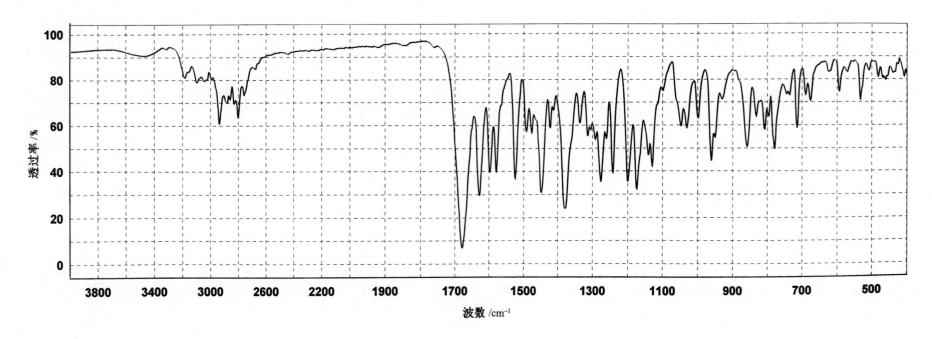

光谱号 1291

中文名：枸橼酸铋钾

英文名：Bismuth Potassium Citrate

分子式：$C_{12}H_{10}BiK_3O_{14}$

药物描述：本品为一种组成不定的含铋复合物。

试样制备：KBr 压片法

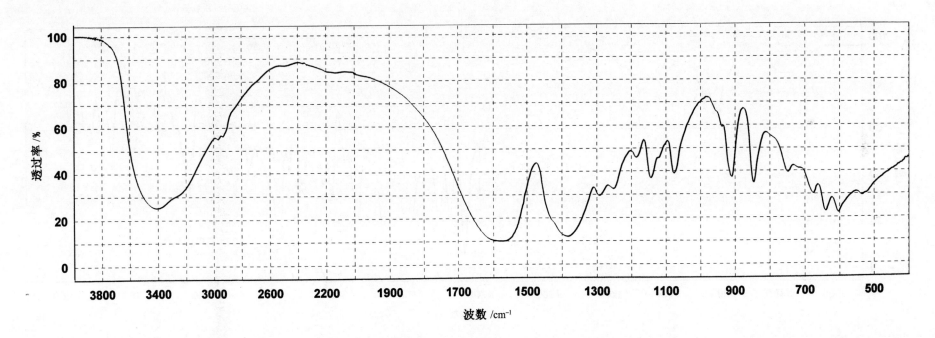

中文名：马来酸桂哌齐特

英文名：Cinepazide Maleate

分子式：C$_{26}$H$_{35}$N$_3$O$_9$

试样制备：KBr 压片法

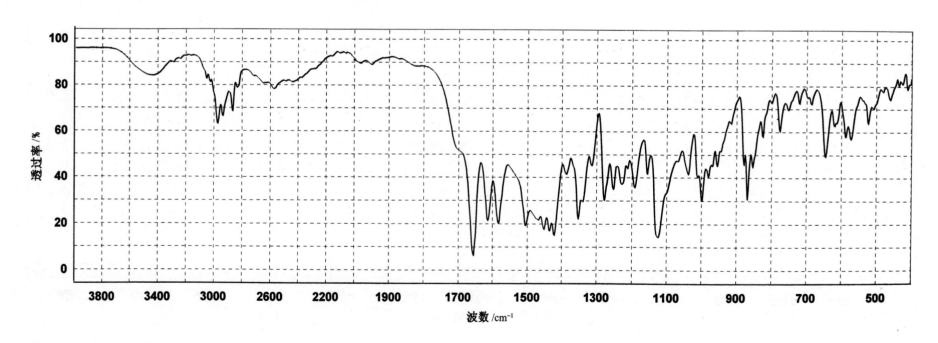

光谱号　1293

中文名：去羟肌苷

英文名：Didanosine

分子式：C$_{10}$H$_{12}$N$_4$O$_3$

试样制备：KBr 压片法

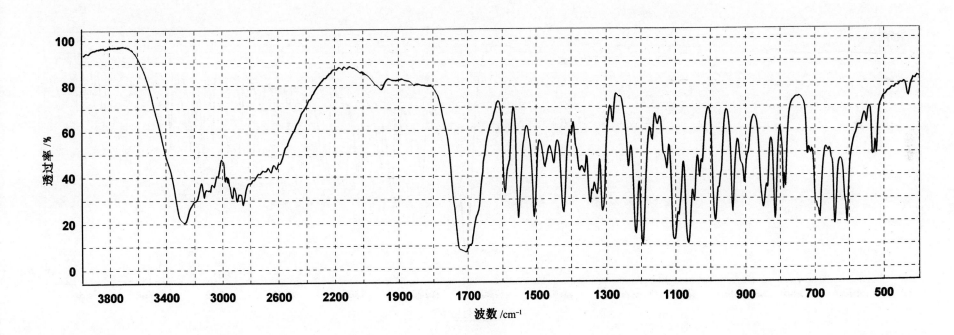

中文名：三苯双脒

英文名：Tribendimidine

分子式：C$_{28}$H$_{32}$N$_6$

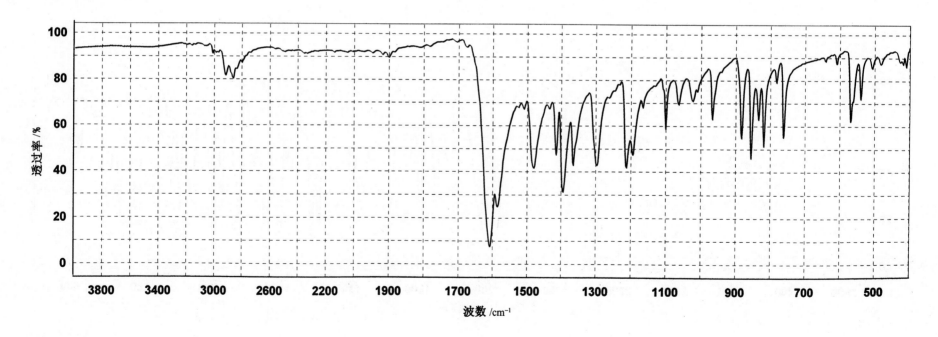

试样制备：KBr 压片法

光谱号　1295

中文名：阿加曲班

英文名：Argatroban

分子式：$C_{23}H_{36}N_6O_5S \cdot H_2O$

试样制备：KBr 压片法

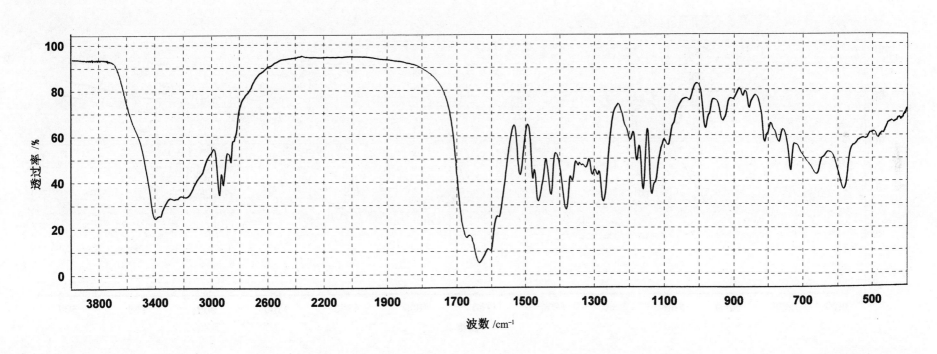

透过率 /%

波数 /cm⁻¹

中文名：果糖二磷酸钠

英文名：Fructose Diphosphate

分子式：C₆H₁₁O₁₂Na₃P₂·8H₂O

试样制备：KBr 压片法

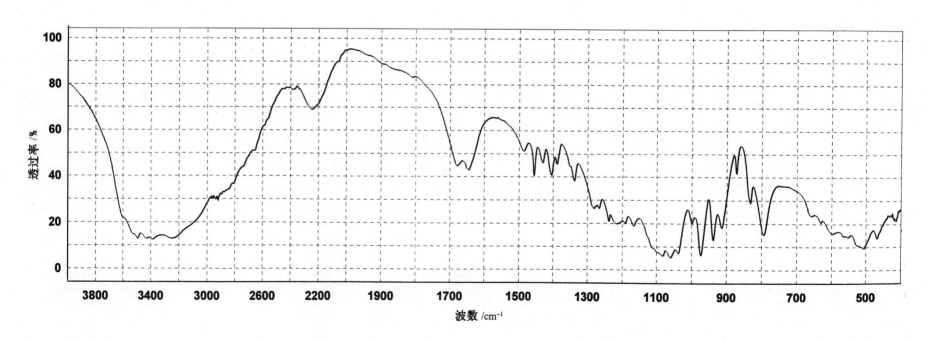

光谱号 1297

中文名：利拉萘酯

英文名：Liranaftate

分子式：C$_{18}$H$_{20}$N$_2$O$_2$S

试样制备：KBr 压片法

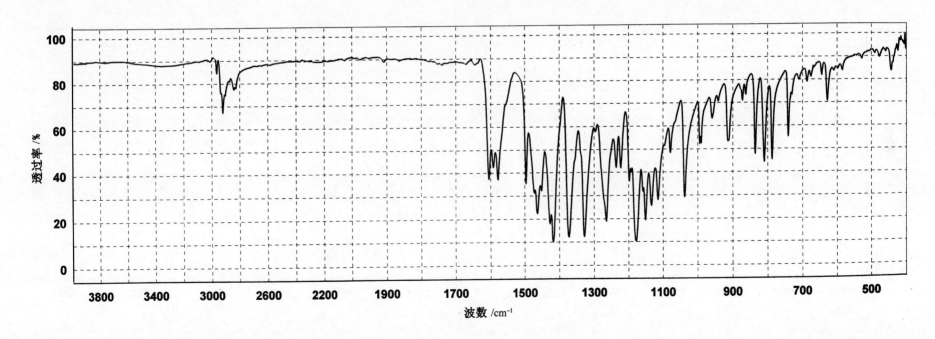

光谱号　1298

中文名：硫酸长春地辛

英文名：Vindesine Sulfate

分子式：C₄₃H₅₅N₅O₇・H₂SO₄

试样制备：KBr 压片法

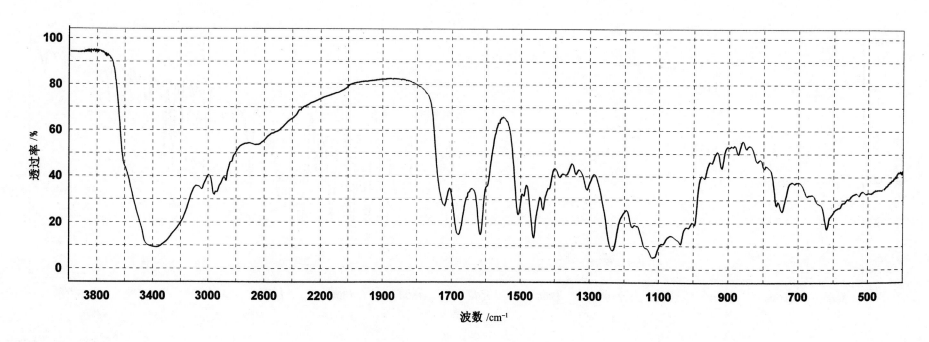

光谱号　1299

中文名：那氟沙星

英文名：Nadifloxacin

分子式：C$_{19}$H$_{21}$FN$_2$O$_4$

试样制备：KBr 压片法

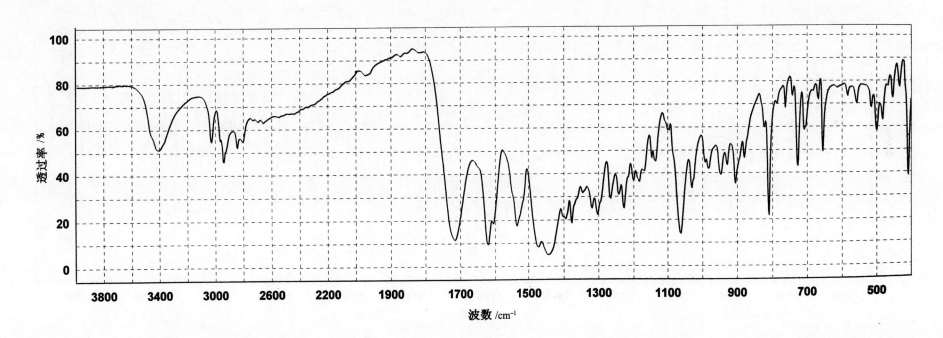

波数 /cm⁻¹

中文名：盐酸尼莫司汀

英文名：Nimustine Hydrochloride

分子式：C₉H₁₃ClN₆O₂·HCl

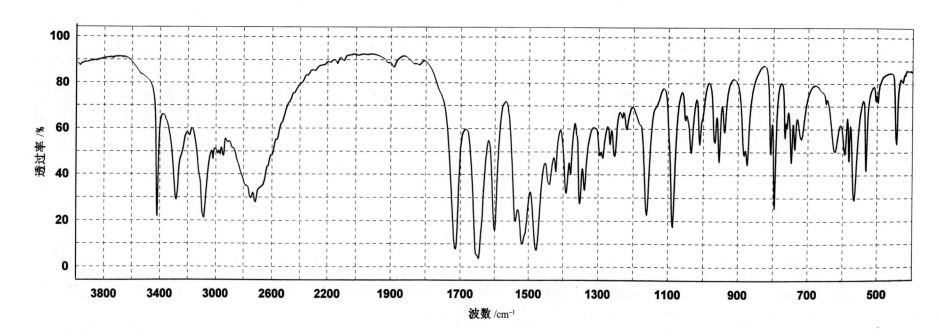

试样制备：KBr 压片法

光谱号　1301

中文名：西尼地平

英文名：Cilnidipine

分子式：C$_{27}$H$_{28}$N$_2$O$_7$

试样制备：KBr 压片法

备注：样品经 80℃减压干燥 4 小时。
Note: Dry at 80℃ in vacuum for 4 hours.

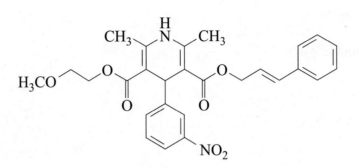

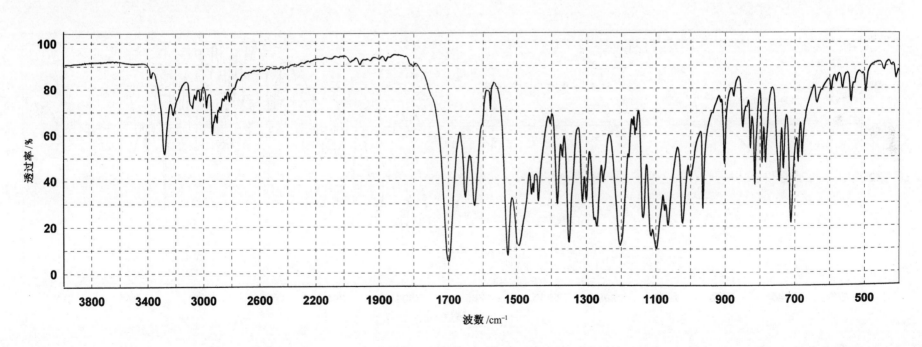

波数 /cm^{-1}

中文名：依地酸钙钠

英文名：Calcium Disodium Edetate

分子式：$C_{10}H_{12}CaN_2Na_2O_8 \cdot 6H_2O$

试样制备：KBr 压片法

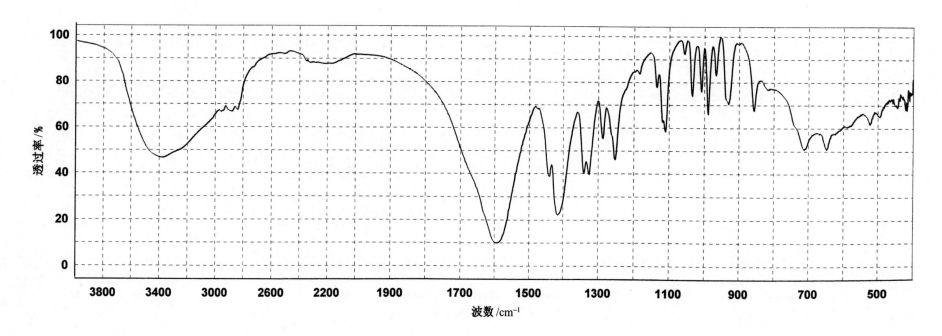

光谱号　1303

中文名：依发韦伦

英文名：Efavirenz

分子式：C$_{14}$H$_9$ClF$_3$NO$_2$

试样制备：KBr 压片法

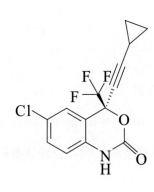

备注：样品常温减压干燥过夜。

Note: Dry at room temperature in vacuum overnight.

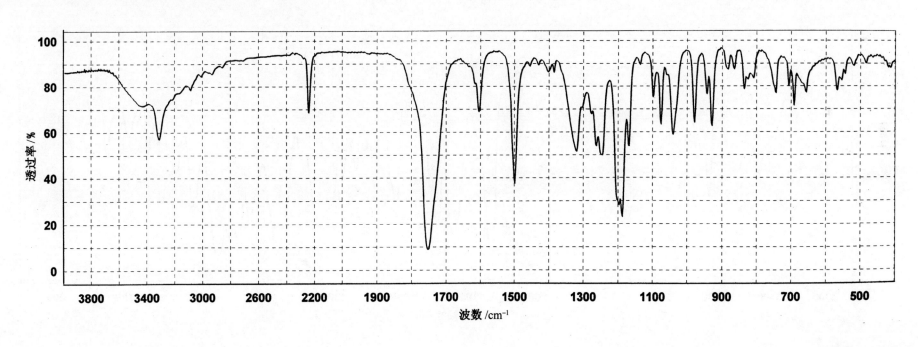

中文名：阿德福韦酯

英文名：Adefovir Dipivoxil

分子式：C$_{20}$H$_{32}$N$_5$O$_8$P

试样制备：液膜法，使用自制的 KBr 片制液膜。

Preparation of sample: Liquid thin film, using a home-made potassium bromide.

备注：取本品约 15mg，加丙酮 0.3ml 使溶解，取溶液数滴滴于空白溴化钾晶片上，红外灯下
挥干溶剂。

Note: Dissolve about 15mg in 0.3ml of acetone, trickle a few drops of the solution into a blank
disc of potassium bromide, evaporate to dryness under infrared light.

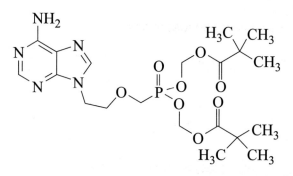

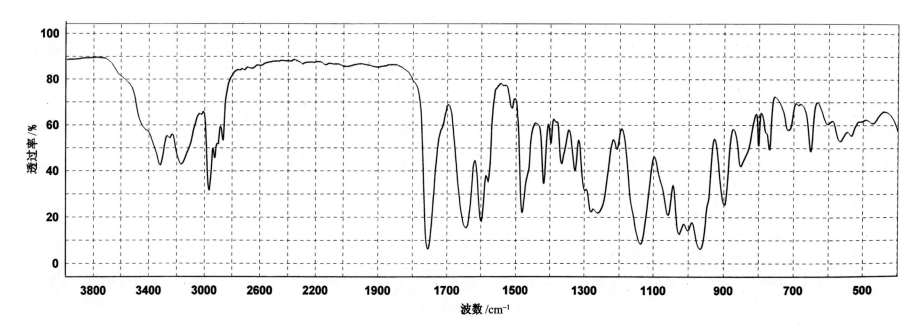

光谱号 1305

中文名：奥美沙坦酯

英文名：Olmesartan Medoxomil

分子式：C$_{29}$H$_{30}$N$_{6}$O$_{6}$

试样制备：KBr 压片法

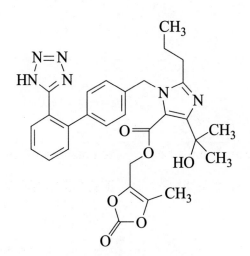

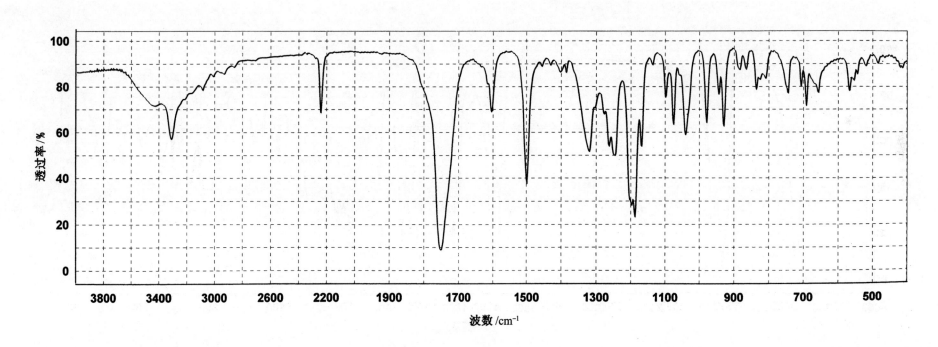

透过率 /%

波数 /cm^{-1}

光谱号 1306

中文名：环戊丙酸雌二醇

英文名：Estradiol Cypionate

分子式：C$_{26}$H$_{36}$O$_3$

试样制备：KBr 压片法

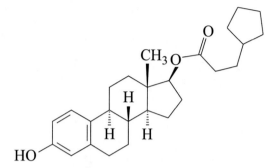

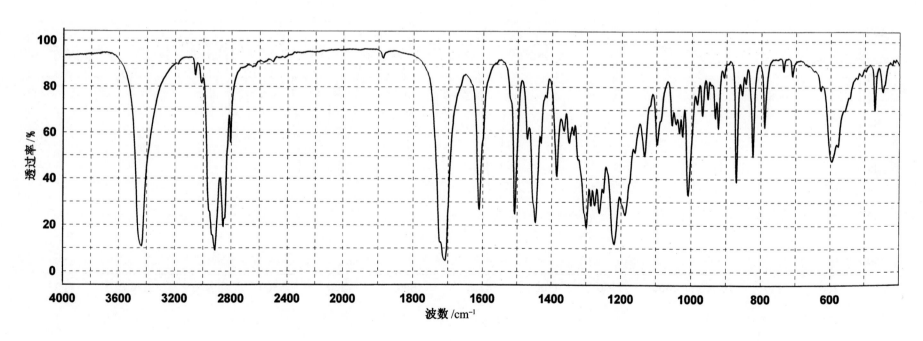

光谱号 1307

中文名：卡培他滨

英文名：Capecitabine

分子式：$C_{15}H_{22}FN_3O_6$

试样制备：KBr 压片法

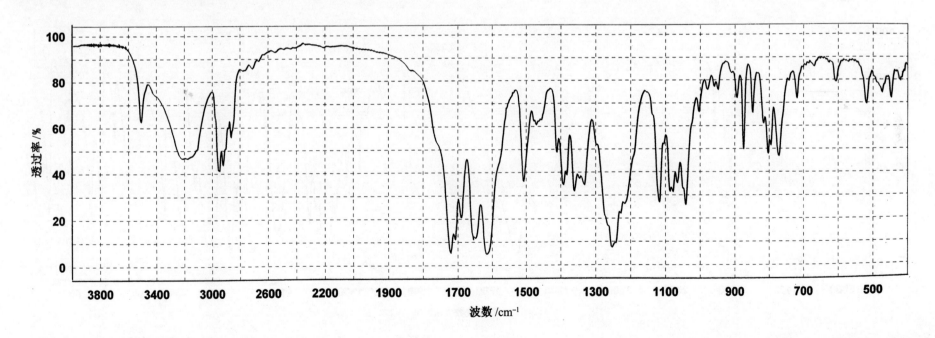

备注：轻微研磨，研磨时间不超过 30 秒。

Note: Grinding slightly, grinding time should be less than 30 seconds.

纵坐标 透过率 /%
横坐标 波数 /cm⁻¹

中文名：去甲斑蝥素

英文名：Norcantharidin

分子式：C$_8$H$_8$O$_4$

试样制备：KBr 压片法

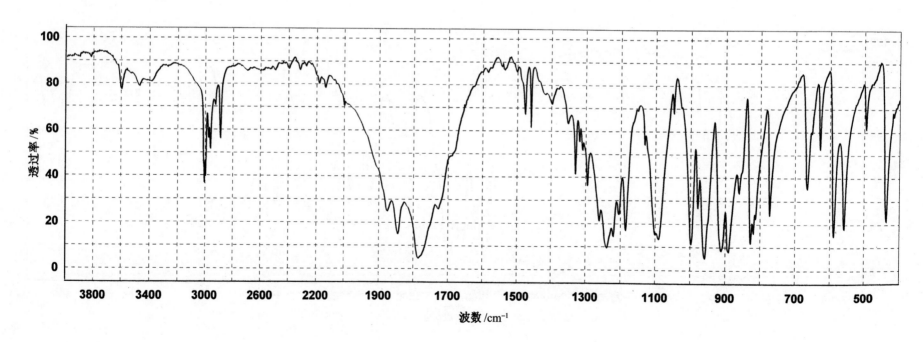

光谱号 1309

中文名：西达本胺

英文名：Chidamide

分子式：C$_{22}$H$_{19}$FN$_4$O$_2$

试样制备：KBr 压片法

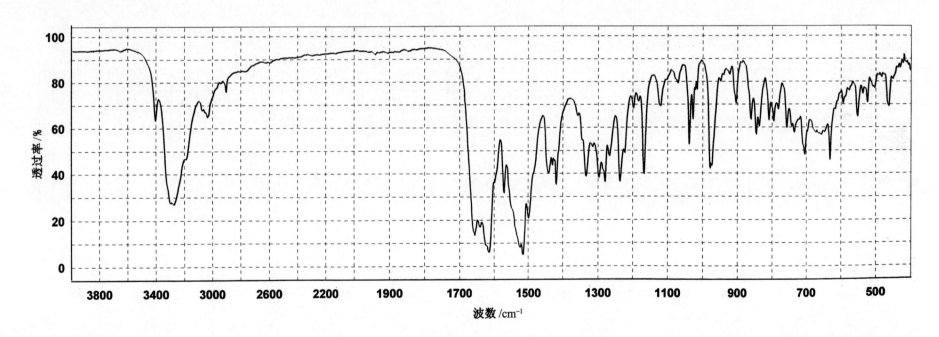

中文名：盐酸雷莫司琼

英文名：Ramosetron Hydrochloride

分子式：C$_{17}$H$_{17}$N$_3$O・HCl

试样制备：KBr 压片法

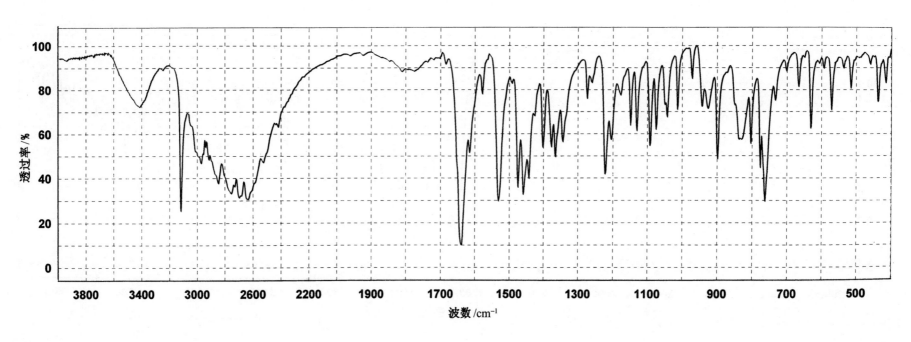

光谱号　1311

中文名：荧光母素

英文名：Fluorane

分子式：C$_{20}$H$_{12}$O$_3$

试样制备：KBr 压片法

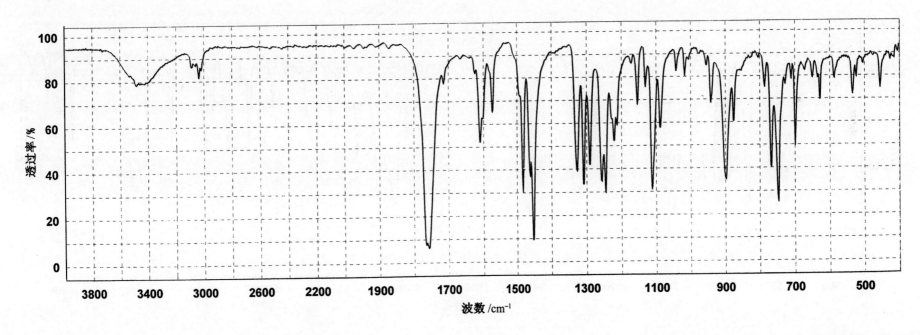

透过率 /%

波数 /cm^{-1}

中文名：盐酸帕吉林

英文名：Pargyline Hydrochloride

分子式：C₁₁H₁₃N·HCl

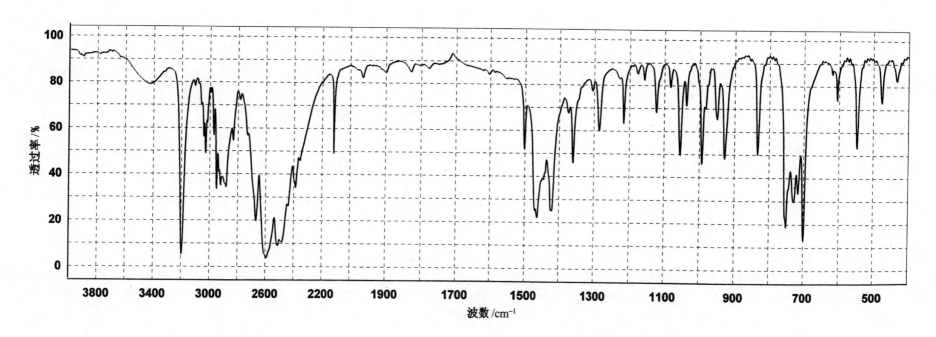

试样制备：KBr 压片法

备注：–20℃避光保存。
Note: Protected from light at –20℃.

中文名：磷酸铝

英文名：Aluminum Phosphate

分子式：AlO₄P

试样制备：KBr 压片法

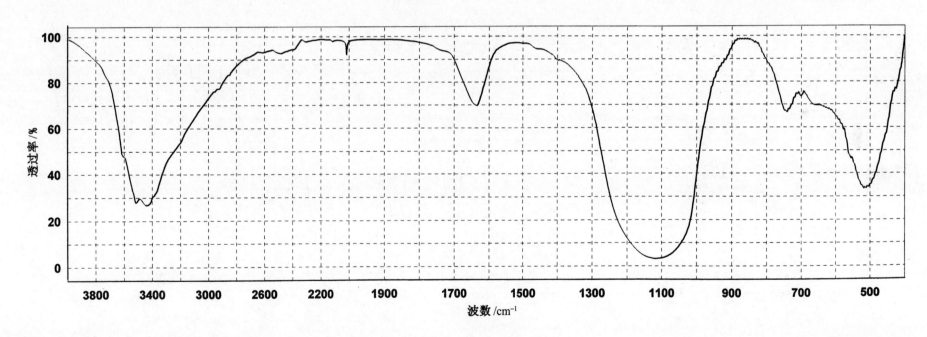

中文名：酒石酸长春瑞滨

英文名：Vinorelbine Tartrate

分子式：C₄₅H₅₄N₄O₈・2C₄H₆O₆

分子式：$C_{45}H_{54}N_4O_8 \cdot 2C_4H_6O_6$

试样制备：KBr 压片法

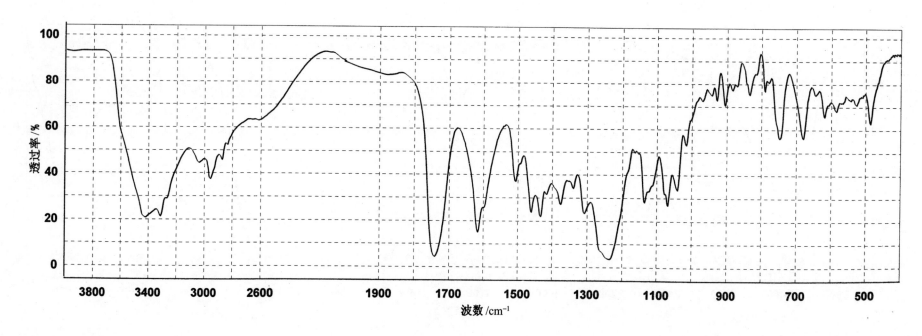

光谱号　1315

中文名：噻苯达唑

英文名：Tiabendazole

分子式：C₁₀H₇N₃S

试样制备：KBr 压片法

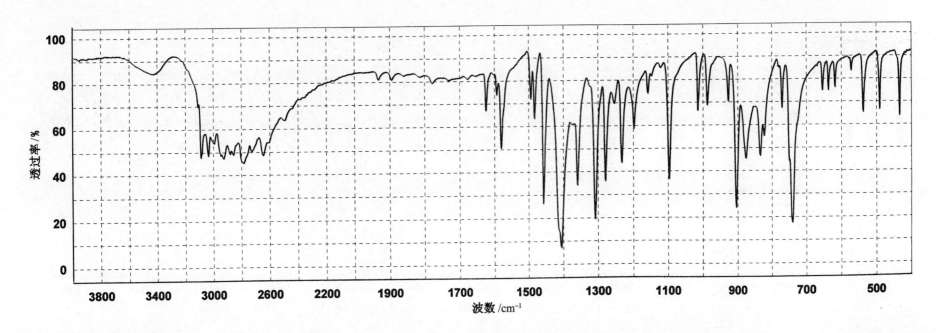

光谱号 1316

中文名：右雷佐生（曾用名：右丙亚胺）

英文名：Dexrazoxane

分子式：$C_{11}H_{16}N_4O_4$

试样制备：KBr 压片法

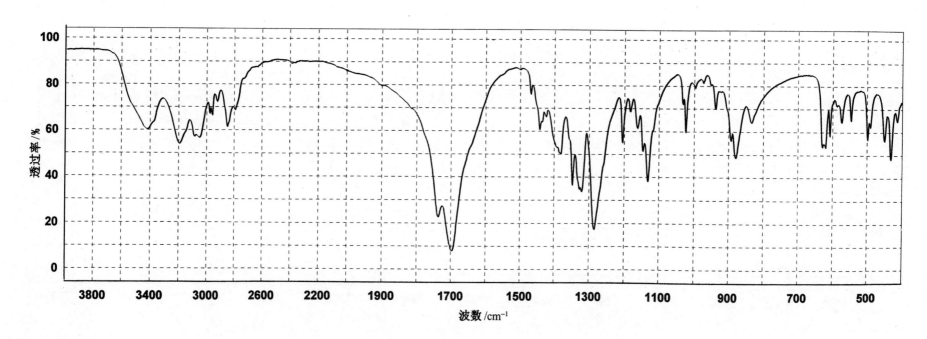

光谱号　1317

中文名：阿雷地平

英文名：Aranidipine

分子式：C₁₉H₂₀N₂O₇

试样制备：KBr 压片法

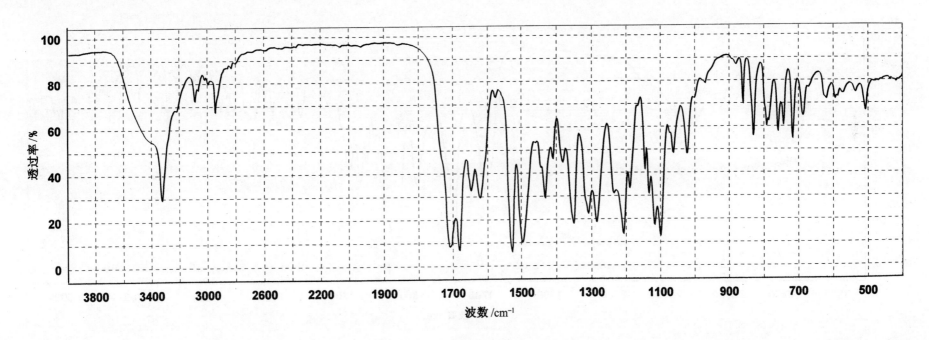

中文名：盐酸莫西沙星

英文名：Moxifloxacin Hydrochloride

分子式：C$_{21}$H$_{24}$FN$_3$O$_4$ · HCl

试样制备：KBr 压片法

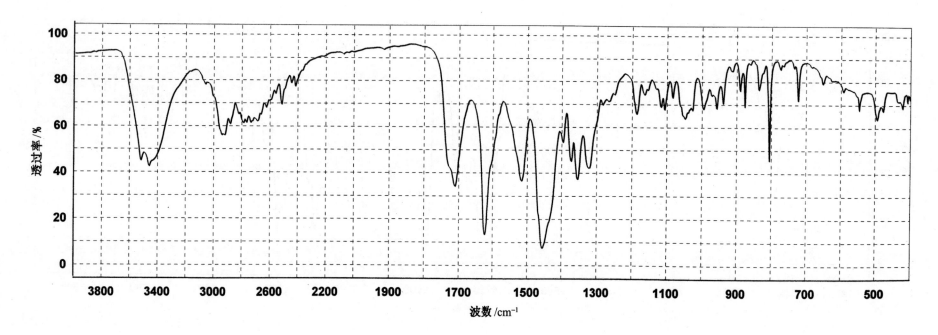

光谱号　1319

中文名：枸橼酸舒芬太尼

英文名：Sufentanil Citrate

分子式：C$_{22}$H$_{30}$N$_2$O$_2$S · C$_6$H$_8$O$_7$

试样制备：KBr 压片法

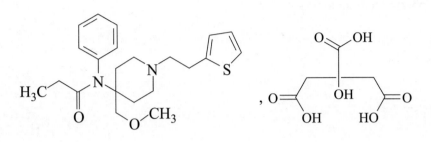

备注：在 105℃干燥 1 小时后测定。

Note: Dry at 105℃ for 1 hour.

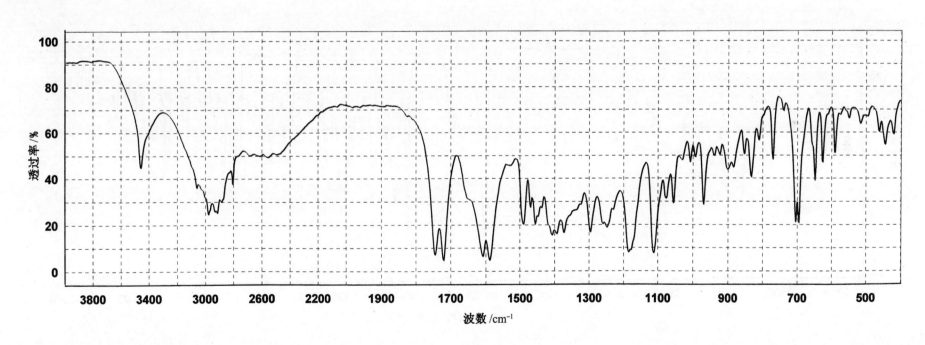

中文名：盐酸氢吗啡酮

英文名：Hydromorphone Hydrochloride

分子式：C$_{17}$H$_{19}$NO$_3$·HCl

试样制备：KBr 压片法

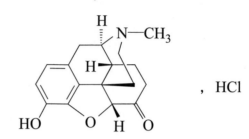

，HCl

备注：在 105℃ 干燥 1 小时后测定。
Note: Dry at 105℃ for 1 hour.

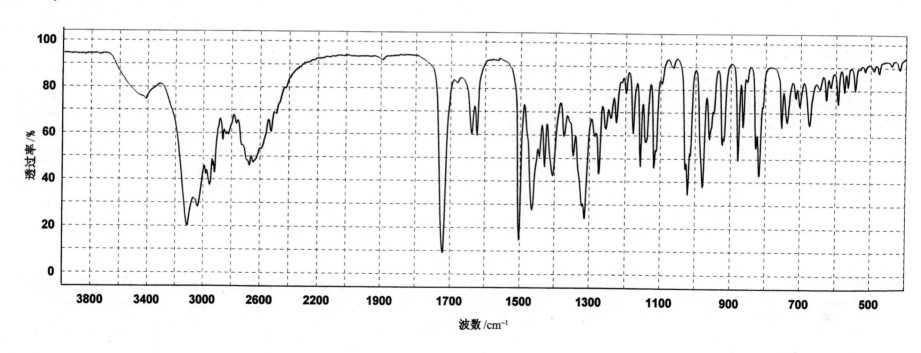

光谱号　1321

中文名: 萘夫西林钠

英文名: Nafcillin Sodium

分子式: C$_{21}$H$_{21}$N$_2$NaO$_5$S · H$_2$O

试样制备: KBr 压片法

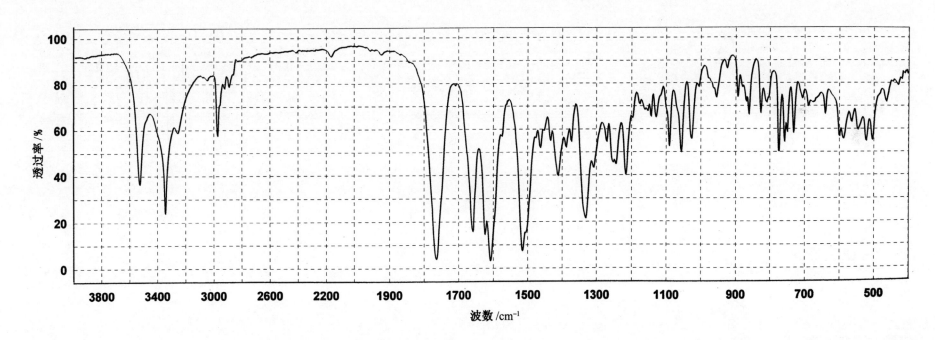

波数 /cm^{-1}

光谱号 1322

中 文 名 索 引

说明：括号中的数字为该药品红外光谱图的光谱号

A

阿德福韦酯（1305）

阿加曲班（1296）

阿雷地平（1318）

阿立哌唑（1291）

阿普唑仑（1271）

氨苄西林钠（1283）

奥美沙坦酯（1306）

B

吡硫翁钠（1272）

苄达赖氨酸（1284）

丙戊酸半钠（1252）

D

达卡巴嗪（1280）

胆酸（1230）

地塞米松棕榈酸酯（1231）

地西他滨（1232）

E

恩替卡韦（1233）

二氮嗪（1234）

二巯丁二钠（1281）

F

夫西地酸钠（1235）

富马酸阿奇霉素（1236）

富马酸喹硫平（1273）

富马酸芦帕他定（1237）

G

甘露醇（1238）

甘油（1268）

更昔洛韦（1266）

谷氨酸（1263）

呱西替柳（1276）

果糖二磷酸钠（1297）

H

环吡酮胺（1258）

环戊丙酸雌二醇（1307）

英 文 名 索 引

说明：括号中的数字为该药品红外光谱图的光谱号

A

Adefovir Dipivoxil（1305）

Adenine（1245）

Alcohol（1290）

Alprazolam（1271）

Aluminum Phosphate（1314）

Ampicillin Sodium（1283）

Aranidipine（1318）

Argatroban（1296）

Aripiprazole（1291）

Asparagine（1274）

Azithromycin Fumarete（1236）

B

Bendazac Lysin（1284）

Benproperine Phosphate（1285）

Bismuth Potassium Citrate（1292）

C

Caffeine（1289）

Calcium Disodium Edetate（1303）

Capecitabine（1308）

Carvedilol（1269）

Chidamide（1310）

Chlormethine Hydrochloride（1255）

Chloroprocaine Hydrochloride（1287）

Cholic Acid（1230）

Ciclopirox Olamine（1258）

Cilastatin Sodium（1253）

Cilnidipine（1302）

Cinepazide Maleate（1293）

Citric Acid（1239）

Clotrimazole（1270）

D

D,L-α-Hydroxymethionine Calcium（1229）

Dacarbazine（1280）

Decitabine（1232）

Dexamethasone Palmitate（1231）

Dexrazoxane（1317）

Diazoxide（1234）

Didanosine（1294）

分 子 式 索 引

说明：括号中的数字为该药品红外光谱图的光谱号

AlO_4P（1314）

C_2H_6O（1290）

$C_3H_5Na_2O_4P$（1251）

$C_3H_8O_3$（1268）

$C_4H_4Na_2O_4S_2 \cdot 3H_2O$（1281）

$C_4H_8N_2O_3 \cdot H_2O$（1274）

C_5H_4NNaOS（1272）

$C_5H_5N_5$（1245）

$C_5H_9NO_4$（1263）

$C_5H_{11}Cl_2N \cdot HCl$（1255）

$C_6H_8O_7 \cdot H_2O$（1239）

$C_6H_{10}N_6O$（1280）

$C_6H_{11}O_{12}Na_3P_2 \cdot 8H_2O$（1297）

$C_6H_{14}N_2O_2 \cdot C_{16}H_{14}N_2O_3$（1284）

$C_6H_{14}O_6$（1238）

$C_6H_{14}O_6$（1278）

$C_8H_7ClN_2O_2S$（1234）

$C_8H_8O_4$（1309）

$C_8H_{10}N_4O_2$（1289）

$C_8H_{12}N_2 \cdot H_3PO_4 \cdot H_2O$（1259）

$C_8H_{12}N_4O_4$（1232）

$C_9H_{13}ClN_6O_2 \cdot HCl$（1301）

$C_9H_{13}N_5O_4$（1266）

$C_9H_{13}NO_2 \cdot C_4H_6O_6$（1262）

$C_9H_{14}N_4O_4$（1240）

$C_{10}H_7N_3S$（1316）

$C_{10}H_{12}CaN_2Na_2O_8 \cdot 6H_2O$（1303）

$C_{10}H_{12}N_4O_3$（1294）

$C_{10}H_{12}N_4O_5S$（1260）

$C_{10}H_{18}CaO_6S_2$（1229）

中文名总索引

说明：括号中的数字为该药品红外光谱图的光谱号

A

阿苯达唑（212，1092）

阿德福韦酯（1305）

阿加曲班（1296）

阿卡波糖（963）

阿克他利（771）

阿雷地平（1318）

阿立哌唑（1291）

阿仑膦酸钠（964）

阿洛西林钠（773）

阿米卡星（20）

阿莫西林（441）

阿莫西林钠（1152）

阿那曲唑（1151）

阿尼西坦（769）

阿普洛尔（774）

阿普唑仑（215，1271）

阿奇霉素（772）

阿嗪米特（967）

阿司咪唑（613）

阿司帕坦（768）

阿司匹林（5）

阿司匹林锌（1107）

阿糖腺苷（968）

阿替洛尔（214）

阿托伐他汀钙（965）

阿维 A（1153）

阿魏酸钠（775）

阿魏酸哌嗪（969）

阿西美辛（770）

阿昔洛韦（213）

阿昔莫司（966）

艾地苯醌（590，1134）

艾司唑仑（63）

安吖啶（607）

安吡昔康（742）

安乃近（159）

安替比林（161）

氨苯蝶啶（413）

氨苯砜（412）

氨苄青霉素三水化合物（658）

氨苄西林钠（411，1283）

氨丁三醇（408）

氨基比林（416）

氨基丁酸（414）

氨基己酸（415）

氨己烯酸（810）

氨甲苯酸（410）

氨甲环酸（409）

氨力农（809）

氨磷汀（1004）

氨鲁米特（417）

氨曲南（1176）

奥氮平（1210）

奥拉米特（1049）

奥拉西坦（1063）

奥美拉唑（675，1050）

奥美拉唑钠（1051）

奥美沙坦酯（1306）

奥沙拉秦钠（858）

奥沙利铂（1209）

奥沙西泮（75）

奥硝唑（1052）

奥扎格雷（674）

奥扎格雷钠（1048）

B

巴比妥（55）

巴氯芬（701）

白消安（935）

斑蝥素（664）

半胱氨酸（711）

半乳糖（710）

棓丙酯（1038）

胞磷胆碱（1000）

胞磷胆碱钠（626，1096）

保泰松（296）

贝美格（704）

贝诺酯（42）

倍他米松（418）

倍他米松二丙酸酯（806）

倍他米松磷酸钠（659）

本芴醇（76）

苯巴比妥（227）

苯巴比妥钠（228）

苯丙氨酸（230，983）

苯丙氨酯（229）

苯丙醇（232）

苯丙酸诺龙（231）

苯丁酸氮芥（226）

苯酚（240）

苯磺阿曲库铵（985）

苯磺顺阿曲库铵（1164）

苯磺酸氨氯地平（790）

苯甲醇（236）

苯甲酸（233）

苯甲酸雌二醇（235）

苯甲酸钠（234）

苯甲酰甲硝唑（984）

苯噻啶（242）

苯替酪胺（241）

苯妥英钠（238）

苯溴马隆（789，1094）

苯扎贝特（787）

苯佐卡因（237）

苯唑西林钠（239）

比沙可啶（35）

吡贝地尔（761）

吡卡酯（186）

吡喹酮（190）

吡拉西坦（185）

吡硫翁钠（1272）

吡罗昔康（188）

吡那地尔（762）

吡诺克辛（763）

吡诺克辛钠（187）

吡哌酸（189）

吡嗪酰胺（191）

扁桃酸（989）

苄达赖氨酸（1284）

苄氟噻嗪（173）

苄星青霉素（172）

别嘌醇（194）

丙氨酸（68，915）

丙泊酚（707）

丙二醇（706）

丙谷胺（67）

丙磺舒（73）

丙硫氧嘧啶（70）

丙硫异烟胺（69）

丙酸倍氯米松（71）

丙酸氟替卡松（916）

丙酸睾酮（72）

丙酸交沙霉素（1115）

丙酸氯倍他索（592）

丙戊酸半钠（1252）

丙戊酸镁（66，1114）

丙戊酸钠（65）

丙戊酰胺（64）

玻璃酸钠（1173）

泊洛沙姆（618）

薄荷脑（891）

布洛芬（85，943）

布美他尼（86）

C

茶苯海明（271）

茶碱（272）

长春胺（705）

长春西汀（588）

常咯啉（435）

穿心莲甙（302）

穿心莲内酯（301，1095）

雌二醇（681）

雌三醇（533）

醋氨苯砜（541）

醋氨己酸锌（888，1103）

醋甘氨酸乙二胺（538）

醋谷胺（539）

醋甲唑胺（1077）

醋氯芬酸（889）

醋羟胺酸（542）

醋酸地塞米松（546）

醋酸氟氢可的松（551）

醋酸氟轻松（550）

醋酸环甲地孕酮（548）

醋酸磺胺米隆（556）

醋酸甲地孕酮（545）

醋酸甲萘氢醌（458）

醋酸甲羟孕酮（160）

醋酸可的松（544）

醋酸赖氨酸（890）

醋酸氯地孕酮（555）

醋酸氯己定（554）

醋酸泼尼松（549）

醋酸泼尼松龙（553）

醋酸氢化可的松（552）

醋酸曲安奈德（547）

醋酸生育酚（455）

醋酸维生素 A（446）

醋酸维生素 E（455）

醋硝香豆素（543）

D

达卡巴嗪（1280）

达那唑（147）

丹皮酚（46）

丹皮酚磺酸钠（47）

单磷酸阿糖腺苷（777，1093）

单硫酸卡那霉素（261）

单氯芬那酸（497）

单硝酸异山梨酯（776）

单盐酸氟西泮（260）

胆酸（1230）

胆影酸（999）

胆甾醇（804）

蛋氨酸（444）

氮甲（118）

地蒽酚（140）

地高辛（139）

地塞米松（741）

地塞米松磷酸钠（141）

地塞米松棕榈酸酯（1231）

地西泮（138）

地西他滨（1232）

碘泊酸钙（521）

碘番酸（522）

碘佛醇（882）

碘苷（520）

碘海醇（1069）

碘解磷定（523）

碘普胺（883，1070）

碘曲仑（748）

碘他拉酸（678）

丁胺卡那霉素（20）

丁苯羟酸（899）

丁二酸洛沙平（686）

丁羟茴醚（687）

丁酸氢化可的松（585）

丁香酚（19）

丁溴东莨菪碱（21）

豆腐果素（961）

豆甾醇（766）

毒毛花甙 K（262）

杜鹃素（168）

度米芬（299）

对氨基水杨酸钠（132）

对乙酰氨基酚（131）

多潘立酮（606）

多索茶碱（941）

多西他赛（1136）

E

鹅去氧胆酸（493）

厄贝沙坦（912）

厄多司坦（1112）

噁丙秦（679）

恩氟烷（807）

恩替卡韦（1233）

二氮嗪（1234）

二氟尼柳（901）

二甲硅油（10）

二甲磺酸阿米三嗪（900）

二甲醚（1109）

二氯醋酸二异丙胺（13）

二羟丙茶碱（12）

二巯丙醇（15）

二巯丁二钠（1281）

二巯丁二酸（14）

二溴甘露醇（16）

二盐酸奎宁（11）

F

法莫替丁（781）

泛喹酮（207）

泛酸钙（208）

泛昔洛韦（956）

泛影酸（209）

放线菌素 D（177）

非布丙醇（246）

非洛地平（794）

非那西丁（247）

非那雄胺（793）

非诺贝特（248）

非诺洛芬钙（249）

非普拉宗（986）

芬布芬（170）

酚磺乙胺（430）

酚酞（429）

粉肌松（123）

奋乃静（243）

夫拉扎勃（39，1146）

夫洛非宁（700）

夫西地酸钠（1235）

呋苄西林钾（178）

呋喃丙胺（179）

呋喃硫胺（183）

呋喃妥因（181）

呋喃唑酮（182）

呋塞米（184）

伏格列波糖（940）

氟胞嘧啶（625）

氟比洛芬（1169）

氟伐他汀钠（1170）

氟康唑（893）

氟罗沙星（799）

氟马西尼（993）

氟米龙（798）

氟尿嘧啶（280）

氟哌啶醇（281）

氟哌利多（624，1171）

氟硼酸盐（717）

氟轻松（800）

氟他胺（797）

福尔可定（531）

福辛普利钠（884）

脯氨酸（436，1041）

辅酶 Q$_{10}$（1046）（曾用名：泛癸利酮）

富马酸阿奇霉素（1236）

富马酸比索洛尔（859）

富马酸喹硫平（1053，1273）

富马酸芦帕他定（1237）

富马酸氯马斯汀（514）

富马酸酮替芬（515）

富马酸亚铁（513）

富马酸异丙吡仑（1211）

G

钆喷酸葡胺（736）

钆双铵（948）

甘氨双唑钠（1129）

甘氨酸（81，929）

甘磷酰芥（83）

甘露醇（84，1238）

甘珀酸钠（80）

甘羟铝（82）

甘油（77，1268）

甘油磷酸钙（78）

甘油磷酸钠（79）

肝素钙（203）

肝素钠（204）

高三尖杉酯碱（420）

膏霉素钾（223）

格列本脲（307）

格列吡嗪（808）

格列喹酮（630，1097）

格列美脲（1085，1175）

格列齐特（629）

格隆溴铵（308）

格鲁米特（309）

葛根素（878）

更昔洛韦（1266）

庚酸炔诺酮（779）

谷氨酸（202，958，1263）

谷氨酸钠（959）

谷氨酸诺氟沙星（960）

谷氨酰胺（895）

谷胱甘肽（765）

呱西替柳（1276）

胱氨酸（419，1036）

甲磺酸加贝酯（1131）

甲磺酸培氟沙星（933）

甲磺酸培高利特（735）

甲磺酸舒他西林（934）

甲磺酸左氧氟沙星（1132）

甲基斑蝥胺（931）

甲基靛玉红（595）

甲基多巴（930）

甲喹酮（115）

甲硫氨酸（1045）

甲硫酸新斯的明（110）

甲硫氧嘧啶（114）

甲氯芬那酸（116）

甲哌占诺（731）

甲巯咪唑（117）

甲硝唑（112）

甲硝唑苯甲酯（113）

甲溴托品（119）

甲氧苄啶（103）

甲氧芳芥（104）

甲氧氟烷（106）

甲氧氯普胺（107）

甲氧沙林（105）

甲状腺素（729）

间苯二酚（206）

交聚维酮（937）

交沙霉素（1135）

角鲨烯（205）

金诺芬（791，1165）

精氨酸（1075）

精氨酸阿司匹林（1225）

酒石酸长春瑞滨（1315）

酒石酸麦角胺（424）

酒石酸美托洛尔（425）

酒石酸托特罗定（1037）

酒石酸昔奈福林（846）

酒石酸唑吡坦（1203）

枸橼酸（263，1239）

枸橼酸铋钾（1292）

枸橼酸芬太尼（266）

枸橼酸钙（796，1168）

枸橼酸氯己定（750）

枸橼酸氯米芬（268）

枸橼酸莫沙必利（991）

枸橼酸喷托维林（267）

枸橼酸舒芬太尼（1320）

枸橼酸他莫昔芬（265）

枸橼酸托瑞米芬（795）

枸橼酸西地那非（990）

枸橼酸乙胺嗪（264）

聚苯乙烯磺酸钙（1226）

K

咖啡因（250，1289）

卡巴胆碱（1117）

卡巴匹林钙（712）

卡比多巴（97）

卡比马唑（95）

卡铂（593）

卡络磺钠（1118）

卡马西平（94）

卡莫氟（713）

卡培他滨（1308）

卡前列甲酯（98）

卡托普利（96）

卡维地洛（714，1269）

坎地沙坦西酯（1147）

糠酸莫米松（814）

考来烯胺（751）

可待因（92）

可可碱（91）

克拉霉素（756）

克拉维酸钾（950）

克林霉素磷酸酯（614）

克罗米通（951）

克霉唑（169，1270）

苦参碱（982）

L

拉呋替丁（1160）

拉米夫定（975）

拉莫三嗪（780）

拉西地平（976）

拉氧头孢钠（1161）

来氟米特（954）

来曲唑（953）

赖氨酸（1071）

赖诺普利（676）

兰索拉唑（708）

榄香烯（1066）

劳拉西泮（1144）

酪氨酸（518，1072）

雷公藤内酯（1073）

雷米普利（1074）

利巴韦林（22）

利福定（952）

利福布汀（1250）

利福喷汀（199，1143）

利福平（198）

利可君（955）

利拉萘酯（1298）

利美索龙（758）

利培酮（759）

利血平（195）

联苯苄唑（666）

联苯双酯（461）

两性霉素 B（176）

亮氨酸（298，987）

邻苯二甲酸羟丙甲纤维素酯（1150）

林旦（977）

磷霉素钙（1080）

磷霉素钠（1251）

磷酸苯丙哌林（579，1285）

磷酸丙吡胺（892）

磷酸伯氨喹（578）

磷酸川芎嗪（1259）

磷酸可待因（577）

磷酸铝（1314）

磷酸萘酚喹（734）

磷酸哌喹（580）

磷酸哌嗪（581）

膦甲酸钠（683）

硫鸟嘌呤（477）

硫喷妥钠（871）

硫普罗宁（872）

硫秋水仙苷（870）

硫酸阿米卡星（1∶1.8）（1079）

硫酸阿托品（487）

硫酸巴龙霉素（483）

硫酸长春地辛（1299）

硫酸长春碱（481）

硫酸长春新碱（480）

硫酸胍乙啶（667）

硫酸卡那霉素（484）

硫酸奎宁（488）

硫酸链霉素（491）

硫酸吗啡（873）

硫酸美芬丁胺（489）

硫酸普拉睾酮钠（874）

硫酸羟氯喹（490）

硫酸氢氯吡格雷（Ⅰ型晶型）（1220）

硫酸氢氯吡格雷（Ⅱ型晶型）（1220）

硫酸庆大霉素（485）

硫酸沙丁胺醇（486）

硫酸双肼屈嗪（482）

硫酸特布他林（668）

硫酸伪麻黄碱（1062）

硫酸小诺米星（479）

硫酸新霉素（492）

硫唑嘌呤（478）

柳氮磺吡啶（620）

六甲蜜胺（692）

咯萘啶（684）

芦丁（174）

卤米松（760）

氯胺 T（500）

氯贝酸铝（495）

氯贝特（494）

氯苯扎利钠（670）

氯氮平（504）

氯氮䓬（505）

氯碘羟喹（506）

氯法齐明（671）

氯琥珀胆碱（496）

氯磺丙脲（508）

氯解磷定（1218）

氯喹（672）

氯雷他定（865）

氯膦酸二钠（866，1219）

氯霉素（507）

氯美扎酮（171）

氯普噻吨（304）

氯噻酮（673）

氯沙坦钾（764）

氯烯雌醚（501）

β－氯腺苷（864）

氯硝柳胺（503）

氯硝西泮（502）

氯氧喹（1217）

氯原酸（863）

氯唑沙宗（499）

氯唑西林钠（200）

罗红霉素（786）

罗舒伐他汀钙（1244）

罗通定（251）

萝巴新（1044）

螺内酯（582）

洛度沙胺氨丁三醇（803）

洛伐他汀（802）

洛莫司汀（300）

洛索洛芬钠（995）

M

马来酸阿奇霉素（1110）

马来酸氨氯地平（908）

马来酸氟伏沙明（907）

马来酸桂哌齐特（1293）

马来酸氯苯那敏（61）

马来酸罗格列酮（906）

马来酸麦角新碱（32）

马来酸曲美布汀（725）

马来酸噻吗洛尔（33）

马来酸替加色罗（1111）

马来酸伊索拉定（905）

马来酸依那普利（587）

马来酸乙酰丙嗪（31）

马洛替酯（34）

马吲哚（691）

吗多明（1240）

吗啡（739）

吗氯贝胺（740）

吗替麦考酚酯（1241）

美罗培南（997）

美洛西林钠（627）

美洛昔康（998）

美沙拉秦（996）

美司钠（1174）

美索巴莫（303）

美他环素（111）

美托洛尔（685）

门冬氨酸（27，913）

门冬氨酸阿奇霉素（904）

门冬氨酸氨氯地平（1081）

门冬氨酸钙（690）

门冬酰胺（1274）

孟鲁司特钠（1242）

咪达唑仑（1084）

咪康唑（276）

咪喹莫特（1167）

咪唑斯汀（1166）

咪唑酸乙酯（275）

米非司酮（162，896，1141）

米格列奈钙（1243）

米力农（749）

米诺地尔（608）

莫匹罗星（845）

莫匹罗星锂（844）

木糖醇（40，1088）

N

那氟沙星（1300）

那格列奈（1142）

那可丁（609）

奈韦拉平（1159）

萘丁美酮（661）

萘啶酸（431）

萘酚喹（662）

萘夫西林钠（1322）

萘磺酸右丙氧芬（1043）

萘莫必利（856）

萘哌地尔（1042）

萘普生（432）

萘普生钠（433）

α-萘乙酸（855）

尼尔雌醇（136）

尼可地尔（134）

尼可刹米（135）

尼麦角林（926）

尼美舒利（598）

尼莫地平（599）

尼群地平（600）

尼索地平（927，1127）

尿囊素（211）

尿素（210）

牛磺酸（44）

诺氟沙星（1202）

P

帕米膦酸二钠（778）

哌泊塞嗪棕榈酸酯（622）

哌喹（274）

哌拉西林（621）

哌拉西林钠（407）

哌西替柳（540）

泮托拉唑钠（1083）

培朵普利（847）

培哚普利叔丁胺盐（1204）

喷昔洛韦（1047）

匹多莫德（693）

匹维溴铵（694）

苹果酸氯波必利（1058）

泼尼松（612，782）

泼尼松龙（284）

扑米酮（62）

葡甲胺（463）

葡醛内酯（467）

葡萄糖（464,702）

葡萄糖酸钙（465）

葡萄糖酸锌（466）

葡萄糖酸亚铁（879）

葡萄糖酸依诺沙星（1221）

普伐他汀钠（860）

普鲁卡因青霉素（511）

普仑司特（1212）

普罗布考（1054）

普罗碘铵（512）

普罗瑞林（1055）

Q

七氟烷（1108）

齐墩果酸（158，1091）

前列地尔（988）

茜草双酯（269）

羟苯丙酯（852）

羟苯丁酯（851）

羟苯磺酸钙（854，1040）

羟苯甲酯（853）

羟苯乙酯（850）

羟布宗（440）

羟丁酸钠（437）

羟基脲（663）

羟甲香豆素（438）

羟甲烟胺（439）

羟萘酸苄芬宁（442）

羟喜树碱（443）

羟乙膦酸钠（1208）

青蒿琥酯（221）

青蒿素（220）

青霉胺（224）

青霉素 V 钾（792）

青霉素钠（222）

氢化可的松（283）

氢化可的松琥珀酸钠（994）

氢氯噻嗪（285）

氢溴酸东莨菪碱（288）

氢溴酸二氢加兰他敏（286）

氢溴酸高乌甲素（290）

氢溴酸后马托品（1172）

氢溴酸加兰他敏（289）

氢溴酸山莨菪碱（287）

氢溴酸烯丙吗啡（291）

氢溴酸右美沙芬（801）

氢溴酸樟柳碱（292）

氰钴铵（449）

秋裂胺（278）

秋水仙碱（277）

巯嘌呤（516）

曲安奈德（603）

曲安西龙（747）

曲尼司特（150，1140）

曲匹布通（148）

曲匹地尔（149）

曲昔派特（1277）

去甲斑蝥素（920，1309）

去羟肌苷（1294）

去氢胆酸（715）

去氧氟尿苷（716）

去乙酰毛花甙（74）

炔雌醇（258）

炔雌醚（1163）

炔诺酮（258）

炔诺孕酮（109）

炔孕酮（617）

R

壬苯醇醚（43）

壬二酸（699）

乳酸钙（254）

乳酸环丙沙星（972）

乳酸诺氟沙星（1154）

乳酸普尼拉明（255）

乳酸依沙吖啶（971）

乳酸左氧氟沙星（970）

乳糖（256）

乳糖酸阿奇霉素（973）

乳糖酸红霉素（257）

瑞巴派特（1067）

瑞格列奈（1068）

S

塞来考昔（1065）

塞替派（530）

噻苯达唑（1316）

噻莫西酸（682）

噻托溴铵（1078）

三苯双脒（1295）

三氮唑核苷（22）

三尖杉酯碱（902）

三磷酸腺苷二钠（903）

三唑仑（586）

色氨酸（156，946）

色甘酸钠（155）

色羟丙钠（157）

沙利度胺（1149）

鲨肝醇（558）

山梨醇（26，1278）

山梨酸（25）

山梨酸钾（688）

芍药苷（752）

麝香草酚（767）

肾上腺素（245）

十一酸睾酮（584）

十一烯酸（17）

十一烯酸锌（18）

石杉碱甲（936）

舒巴坦钠（509）

舒必利（510）

舒林酸（877）

舒马普坦（876）

双环醇（1113）

双氯非那胺（54）

双氯芬酸二乙胺（697）

双氯芬酸钾（698）

双氯芬酸钠（53）

双吗仑（49）

双嘧达莫（557）

双喃氟啶（52）

双羟萘酸奥克太尔（1286）

双羟萘酸噻嘧啶（51）

双氢青蒿素（696）

双炔失碳酯（50）

水飞蓟素（56）

水杨酸（57）

水杨酸毒扁豆碱（58）

水杨酸二乙胺（703）

水杨酸甲酯（709）

水杨酸镁（60）

水杨酸咪唑（589）

水杨酸钠（59）

顺铂（297）

丝氨酸（133，917）

丝裂霉素（918）

司可巴比妥钠（137）

司莫司汀（1119）

司帕沙星（921）

司坦唑醇（597）

四（甲氧异丁腈）络铜（Ⅰ）氟硼酸盐（717）

四环素（122）

松醇（225）

苏氨酸（175，957）

羧苄西林钠（529）

羧甲司坦（885）

T

他扎罗汀（919，1116）

他唑巴坦（1260）

酞丁安（427）

酞磺胺噻唑（428）

糖精钠（576）

特非那定（244）

替比夫定（1213）

替勃龙（1215）

替加氟（861）

替考拉宁（1214）

替米沙坦（1057）

替莫唑胺（1216）

替尼泊苷（1056）

替硝唑（665）

天麻素（914）

酮苯丙氨酸钙（1222）

酮康唑（677）

酮亮氨酸钙（1223）

酮咯酸氨丁三醇（1224）

酮洛芬（517）

头孢氨苄（128，1090）

头孢丙烯（1120）

头孢泊肟酯（1124）

头孢地尼（1122）

头孢地秦钠（922）

头孢呋辛钠（721）

头孢呋辛酯（923）

头孢克洛（720）

头孢克肟（719）

头孢拉定（722）

头孢硫脒（924）

头孢美唑钠（1125）

头孢孟多酯钠（125）

头孢尼西钠（1121）

头孢哌酮钠（126，1089）

头孢羟氨苄（596）

头孢曲松钠（124）

头孢噻吩钠（129）

头孢噻肟钠（130）

头孢他啶（718）

头孢替唑钠（1126）

头孢西丁钠（1123）

头孢唑林钠（127）

头孢唑肟钠（723）

土大黄甙（23）

土霉素（24）

托吡卡胺（746，1267）

托吡酯（949）

托美丁钠（945）

托西酸舒他西林（1261）

W

维 A 酸（445）

维胺酸（849）

维胺酯（1207）

维库溴铵（848）

维生素 B_1（1205）

维生素 B_2（447）

维生素 B_6（448）

维生素 B_{12}（449）

维生素 C（450）

维生素 C 钙（451）

维生素 C 钠（1039）

维生素 D_2（452）

维生素 D_3（453）

维生素 E（1206）

维生素 K_1（456）

维生素 U（459）

伪麻黄碱（604）

乌苯美司（911）

乌芬那酯（623）

乌拉地尔（910）

乌洛托品（45）

乌司他丁（909）

无水葡萄糖（702）

五氟利多（41）

戊四氮（727）

戊酸倍他米松（89）

戊酸雌二醇（90）

戊酮酸钙（88）

X

西吡氯铵（947）

西达本胺（1310）

西洛他唑（754）

西咪替丁（142）

西尼地平（1302）

西沙必利（753）

西司他丁钠（1253）

昔萘酸沙美特罗（1162）

喜树碱（857）

α－细辛脑（619）

腺苷（886）

腺苷钴胺（887）

腺嘌呤（1245）

香草醛（1001）

消旋卡多曲（1005）

消旋羟蛋氨酸钙（1229）

消旋山莨菪碱（811）

硝苯地平（469）

硝呋醛（180）

硝呋太尔（868）

硝普钠（1061）

硝酸硫胺（476）

硝酸毛果芸香碱（472）

硝酸咪康唑（474）

硝酸士的宁（869）

硝酸一叶萩碱（471）

硝酸异山梨酯（473）

硝酸益康唑（475）

硝西泮（470）

缬氨酸（559，1076）

缬沙坦（1227）

辛伐他汀（962）

熊去氧胆酸（534）

溴吡斯的明（527）

溴丙胺太林（525）

溴醋己烷雌酚（528）

溴夫定（880）

溴甲贝那替秦（680）

溴莫普林（881）

溴新斯的明（526）

Y

亚胺醌（144）

亚胺培南（1254）

亚甲蓝（143）

亚硫酸氢钾苯丁酮（145）

亚硫酸氢钠甲萘醌（457）

亚叶酸钙（737）

亚乙双半胱氨酸（695）

烟酸（422）

烟酸生育酚（454）

烟酸维生素 E（454）

烟酸占替诺（660）

烟酰胺（421）

盐酸阿夫唑嗪（1087）

盐酸阿米洛利（828）

盐酸阿米替林（360）

盐酸阿扑吗啡（359）

盐酸阿普林定（829）

盐酸阿糖胞苷（361）

盐酸阿扎司琼（1019）

盐酸艾司洛尔（635，1264）

盐酸安非拉酮（823）

盐酸安他唑啉（348）

盐酸安西他滨（644）

盐酸氨基葡萄糖（652）

盐酸氨溴索（839，1102）

盐酸胺碘酮（382）

盐酸昂丹司琼（832）

盐酸奥布卡因（316）

盐酸奥普力农（1246）

盐酸奥昔布宁（1032）

盐酸奥昔非君（394）

盐酸半胱氨酸（333，816）

盐酸贝凡洛尔（1182）

盐酸贝那普利（836）

盐酸贝那替秦（321）

盐酸贝尼地平（1183）

盐酸倍他司汀（838）

盐酸苯丙醇胺（364）

盐酸苯海拉明（365）

盐酸苯海索（366）

盐酸苯环壬酯（1021）

盐酸苯乙双胍（363）

盐酸吡格列酮（1192）

盐酸吡硫醇（356）

盐酸苄达明（355）

盐酸苄普地尔（1018）

盐酸苄丝肼（1017）

盐酸表柔比星（1022）

盐酸丙卡特罗（637）

盐酸丙米嗪（638）

盐酸丙哌维林（1009）

盐酸布比卡因（324）

盐酸布桂嗪（315）

盐酸布替萘芬（1185）

盐酸川芎嗪（319，1098）

盐酸达克罗宁（341）

盐酸大观霉素（1007）

盐酸氮芥（390，1255）

盐酸地巴唑（336）

盐酸地尔硫䓬（337）

盐酸地芬尼多（338）

盐酸地芬诺酯（339）

盐酸地拉䓬（340）

盐酸地匹福林（335）

盐酸丁丙诺啡（633）

盐酸丁卡因（314）

盐酸丁咯地尔（813，1177）

盐酸丁螺环酮（1178）

盐酸多巴胺（345）

盐酸多巴酚丁胺（346）

盐酸多奈哌齐（1188）

盐酸多柔比星（1015）

盐酸多塞平（347）

盐酸多沙普仑（643，1256）

盐酸多西环素（386）

盐酸二苯美仑（632）

盐酸二甲双胍（631）

盐酸二氢埃托啡（313，1179）

盐酸二氧丙嗪（322）

盐酸伐昔洛韦（1013）

盐酸法舒地尔（1195）

盐酸芬氟拉明（354）

盐酸酚苄明（384）

盐酸酚妥拉明（353）

盐酸氟奋乃静（378）

盐酸氟桂利嗪（379）

盐酸氟西泮（377）

盐酸氟西汀（837）

盐酸戈洛帕米（815）

盐酸格拉司琼（1027）

盐酸关附甲素（645）

盐酸海索那林（383）

盐酸环丙沙星（647，1100）

盐酸环仑特罗（362）

盐酸黄酮哌酯（1031）

盐酸吉西他滨（1014）

盐酸甲砜霉素甘氨酸酯（1247）

盐酸甲基麻黄碱（330）

盐酸甲氯芬酯（331）

盐酸甲氧明（329）

盐酸甲氧那明（1086）

盐酸金刚烷胺（369）

盐酸金刚乙胺（1196）

盐酸金霉素（370）

盐酸精氨酸（406）

盐酸肼屈嗪（371）

盐酸卡波罗孟（639）

盐酸卡尼汀（328）

盐酸卡替洛尔（817）

盐酸可卡因（326）

盐酸可乐定（327）

盐酸克林霉素（352）

盐酸克林霉素棕榈酸酯（757）

盐酸克仑特罗（351）

盐酸奎宁（373，1101）

盐酸喹那普利（1200）

盐酸赖氨酸（399，1035）

盐酸雷甲氨酯（400）

盐酸雷莫司琼（1311）

盐酸雷尼替丁（401）

盐酸利多卡因（357）

盐酸林可霉素（833）

盐酸硫胺（654）

盐酸硫必利（1033）

盐酸硫利达嗪（1034）

盐酸芦氟沙星（827）

盐酸氯胺酮（393）

盐酸氯丙那林（655）

盐酸氯丙嗪（391）

盐酸氯环利嗪（656）

盐酸氯己定（380）

盐酸氯米帕明（842）

盐酸氯哌斯汀（392）

盐酸氯普鲁卡因（1287）

盐酸罗沙替丁醋酸酯（1248）

盐酸罗通定（834）

盐酸洛贝林（318，1197）

盐酸洛非西定（1025）

盐酸洛美沙星（650）

盐酸洛哌丁胺（649，1257）

盐酸麻黄碱（387）

盐酸马普替林（634）

盐酸吗啡（344）

盐酸吗啉胍（343）

盐酸美他环素（1026）

盐酸美西律（381）

盐酸咪达普利（1024）

盐酸米安色林（1191）

盐酸米诺环素（825）

盐酸米托蒽醌（824）

盐酸莫雷西嗪（651）

盐酸莫索尼定（1029）

盐酸莫西沙星（1319）

盐酸纳洛酮（646）

盐酸纳曲酮（1194）

盐酸奈福泮（367）

盐酸萘甲唑啉（385）

盐酸萘替芬（1030）

盐酸尼卡地平（334）

盐酸尼莫司汀（1301）

盐酸帕吉林（1313）

盐酸帕罗西汀（831）

盐酸哌甲酯（374）

盐酸哌仑西平（648）

盐酸哌替啶（376）

盐酸哌唑嗪（375）

盐酸普鲁卡因（397）

盐酸普鲁卡因胺（398）

盐酸普罗帕酮（395）

盐酸普萘洛尔（396）

盐酸羟苄唑（388）

盐酸羟甲唑啉（653）

盐酸青藤碱（1023）

盐酸氢吗啡酮（1321）

盐酸曲马朵（641）

盐酸曲美他嗪（1189）

盐酸曲普利啶（1190）

盐酸去甲伪麻黄碱（818）

盐酸去氯羟嗪（820）

盐酸去氧肾上腺素（819）

盐酸柔红霉素（323）

盐酸瑞芬太尼（1288）

盐酸塞利洛尔（843，1201）

盐酸噻氯匹定（640）

盐酸赛庚啶（404）

盐酸赛克利嗪（403）

盐酸赛洛唑啉（657，1279）

盐酸三氟拉嗪（317）

盐酸舍曲林（835）

盐酸舒托必利（1282）

盐酸司来吉兰（821）

盐酸四环素（332）

盐酸索他洛尔（1028，1199）

盐酸坦洛新（830）

盐酸特比萘芬（840，1198）

盐酸特拉唑嗪（841）

盐酸头孢吡肟（1184）

盐酸头孢他美酯（1011）

盐酸头孢替安（822）

盐酸土霉素（1064）

盐酸托泊替康（1020）

盐酸托哌酮（342，1099）

盐酸妥拉唑林（1193）

盐酸妥洛特罗（358）

盐酸万古霉素（1180）

盐酸维拉帕米（389）

盐酸伪麻黄碱（642）

盐酸文拉法辛（1008，1265）

盐酸乌拉地尔（1181）

盐酸戊乙奎醚（1186）

盐酸西布曲明（1016）

盐酸西替利嗪（826）

盐酸小檗碱（320）

盐酸溴己新（402）

盐酸伊托必利（1187）

盐酸依普拉酮（368）

盐酸乙胺丁醇（311）

盐酸乙基吗啡（312）

盐酸乙哌立松（812）

盐酸异丙嗪（350）

盐酸异丙肾上腺素（349）

盐酸罂粟碱（405）

盐酸右异可利定（1010）

盐酸组氨酸（372）

盐酸左布诺洛尔（636）

盐酸左旋咪唑（325）

盐酸左氧氟沙星（1012）

氧氟沙星（1003）

叶酸（93）

伊班膦酸钠（939）

伊拉地平（738）

伊曲康唑（938）

伊索昔康（151）

依地酸二钠（978）

依地酸钙钠（252，1303）

依发韦伦（1304）

依立雄胺（1006）

依那普利拉（1157）

依诺沙星（282）

依帕司他（1249）

依普黄酮（616，745）

依他尼酸（196）

依他尼酸钠（197）

依替膦酸二钠（1158）

依托泊苷（615）

依托度酸（974）

依托芬那酯（1155）

依托红霉素（36）

依托咪酯（253）

依西美坦（1156）

乙胺硫脲（897）

乙胺嘧啶（3）

乙胺锌（583）

乙醇（1290）

乙琥胺（4）

乙水杨胺（1）

N–乙酰–L–酪氨酸（1105）

N–乙酰–L–色氨酸（1104）

乙酰半胱氨酸（7）

乙酰谷酰胺（539）（曾用名：醋谷胺）

乙酰胡椒甲胺（8）

乙酰水杨酸孕烯诺龙（6）

乙酰天麻素（898）

乙酰唑胺（9）

乙氧苯柳胺（1106）

乙氧黄酮（2）

异丙安替比林（942）

异丁司特（743）

异氟烷（744，1139）

异环磷酰胺（1138）

异亮氨酸（165，894）

异山梨醇（1137）

异维 A 酸（944）

异戊巴比妥（163）

异戊巴比妥钠（164）

异烟肼（166）

益多酯（426）

吲达帕胺（192，1275）

吲哚布芬（1145）

吲哚菁绿（611）

吲哚洛尔（610）

吲哚美辛（193）

荧光母素（1312）

荧光素钠（273）

硬脂酸红霉素（468）

右苯丙胺（788）

右雷佐生（曾用名：右丙亚胺）（1317）

鱼腥草素钠（153）

愈创甘油醚（524）

月桂氮草酮（48）

孕二烯酮（724）

孕三烯酮（925）

Z

樟脑（535）

樟脑磺酸钠（537）

樟脑酸（536）

栀子苷（992）

重酒石酸胆碱（295）

重酒石酸间羟胺（294，1262）

重酒石酸去甲肾上腺素（293）

紫杉醇（875）

棕榈氯霉素（A 型）（37）

棕榈氯霉素（B 型）（38）

棕榈哌泊塞（622）

棕榈酸（862）

组氨酸（785，981）

左谷酰胺（201）

左甲状腺素钠（928）

左卡尼汀（591）

左炔诺孕酮（726）

左旋多巴（87）

左氧氟沙星（1128）

佐匹克隆（755）

英文名总索引

说明：括号中的数字为该药品红外光谱图的光谱号

A

Acarbose（963）

Aceclofenac（889）

Acedapsone（541）

Acegastrodine（898）

Aceglutamide（539）

Acemetacin（770）

Acenocoumarol（543）

Acepromazine Maleate（31）

Acetazolamide（9）

Acetohydroxamic Acid（542）

Acetylcysteine（7）

N-Acetyl-L-tryptophan（1104）

N-Acetyl-L-tyrosine（1105）

Acetylsalicylic Acid（5）

Aciclovir（213）

Acipimox（966）

Acitretin（1153）

Actarit（771）

Adefovir Dipivoxil（1305）

Adenine（1245）

Adenosine（886）

Adenosine Cyclophosphate（219）

Adenosine Disodium Triphosphate（903）

Adipiodone（999）

Adrenaline（245）

Alanine（68，915）

Albendazole（212，1092）

Alcohol（1290）

Alendronate Sodium（964）

Alfuzosin Hydrochloride（1087）

Allantoin（211）

Allopurinol（194）

Almitrine Bismesylate（900）

Alprazolam（215，1271）

Alprenolol（774）

Alprostadil（988）

Altretamine（692）

Aluminum Clofibrate（495）

Aluminum Phosphate（1314）

Amantadine Hydrochloride（369）

Ambroxol Hydrochloride（839，1102）

Amfepramone Hydrochloride（823）

Amidopyrine（416）

Amifostine（1004）

Amikacin（20）

Amikacin Sulfate（1079）

Amiloride Hydrochloride（828）

Aminobutyric Acid（414）

Aminocaproic Acid（415）

Aminoglutethimide（417）

Aminomethylbenzoic Acid（410）

Aminophenazone（416）

Amiodarone Hydrochloride（382）

Amitriptyline Hydrochloride（360）

Amlodipine Aspartate（1081）

Amlodipine Besylate（790）

Amlodipine Maleate（908）

Amlodipine Mesylate（1133）

Amobarbital（163）

Amobarbital Sodium（164）

Amoxicillin（441）

Amoxicillin Sodium（1152）

Amphotericin B（176）

Ampicillin Sodium（411，1283）

Ampicillin Trihydrate（658）

Ampiroxicam（742）

Amrinone（809）

Amsacrine（607）

Anastrozole（1151）

Ancitabine Hydrochloride（644）

Andrographolide（301，1095）

Anethol Trithione（270）

Anhydrous Glucose（702）

Aniracetam（769）

Anisodamine Hydrobromide（287）

Anisodine Hydrobromide（292）

Anorethindrane Dipropionate（50）

Antazoline Hydrochloride（348）

Apomorphine Hydrochloride（359）

Aprindine Hydrochloride（829）

Aranidipine（1318）

Argatroban（1296）

Arginine（1075）

Arginine Aspirin（1225）

Arginine Monohydrochloride（406）

Aripiprazole（1291）

Artemether（519）

Artemisinin（220）

Artesunate（221）

α-Asarone（619）

Ascorbic Acid（450）

Asparagine（1274）

Aspartame（768）

Aspartic Acid（27，913）

Aspirin（5）

Aspirin Zinc（1107）

Astemizole（613）

Atenolol（214）

Atorvastatin Calcium（965）

Atracurium Besilate（985，1164）

Atropine Methylbromide（119）

Atropine Sulfate（487）

Auranofin（791，1165）

Azasetron Hydrochloride（1019）

Azathioprine（478）

Azelaic Acid（699）

Azintamide（967）

Azithromycin（772）

Azithromycin Aspartate（904）

Azithromycin Fumarete（1236）

Azithromycin Lactobionate（973）

Azithromycin Maleate（1110）

Azlocillin Sodium（773）

Aztreonam（1176）

B

Baclofen（701）

Barbital（55）

Batilol（558）

Beclometasone Dipropionate（71）

Bemegride（704）

Benactyzine Hydrochloride（321）

Benazepril Hydrochloride（836）

Bendazac Lysin（1284）

Bendazol Hydrochloride（336）

Bendroflumethiazide（173）

Benflumetol（76）

Benidipine Hydrochloride（1183）

Benorilate（42）

Benproperine Phosphate（579，1285）

Benserazid Hydrochloride（1017）

Bentiromide（241）

Benzathine Benzylpenicillin（172）

Benzbromarone（789，1094）

Benzhexol Hydrochloride（366）

Benzocaine（237）

Benzoic Acid（233）

Benzoyl Peroxide（602）

Benzoylmetronidazole（984）

Benzydamine Hydrochloride（355）

Benzyl Alcohol（236）

Benzylpenicillin Potassium（223）

Benzylpenicillin Sodium（222）

Bephenium Hydroxynaphthoate（442）

Bepridil Hydrochloride（1018）

Berberine Hydrochloride（320）

Betahistine Hydrochloride（838）

Betamethasone（418）

Betamethasone Dipropionate（806）

Betamethasone Sodium Phosphate（659）

Betamethasone Valerate（89）

Bevantolol Hydrochloride（1182）

Bezafibrate（787）

Bicyclol（1113）

Bifemelane Hydrochloride（632）

Bifendate（461）

Bifonazole（666）

Bimolanl（49）

Bisacodyl（35）

Bismuth Potassium Citrate（1292）

Bisoprolol Fumarate（859）

Brivudine（880）

Brodimoprim（881）

Bromhexine Hydrochloride（402）

Bucinnazine Hydrochloride（315）

Bufexamac（899）

Buflomedil Hydrochloride（813，1177）

Bumetanide（86）

Bupivacaine Hydrochloride（324）

Buprenorphine Hydrochloride（633）

Buspirone Hydrochloride（1178）

Busulfan（935）

Butenafine Hydrochloride（1185）

Butylated Hydroxyanisole（687）

Butylparaben（851）

C

Caffeine（250，1289）

Calcium Ascorbate（451）

Calcium Aspartate（690）

Calcium Citrate（796）

Calcium Disodium Edetate（1303）

Calcium Disodium（252）

Calcium Dobesilate（854，1040）

Calcium Folinate（737）

Calcium Gluconate（465）

Calcium Glycerophosphate（78）

Calcium Iopodate（521）

Calcium Lactate（254）

Calcium Levulinate（88）

Calcium Pantothenate（208）

Calcium Polystyrene Sulphonate（1226）

Camphor（535）

Chloroxoquinoline（1217）

Chlorphenamine Maleate（61）

Chlorpromazine Hydrochloride（391）

Chlorpropamide（508）

Chlorprothixene（304）

Chlortalidone（673）

Chlortetracycline Hydrochloride（370）

Chlorzoxazone（499）

Cholesterol（804）

Cholestyramine（751）

Cholic Acid（1230）

Choline Bitartrate（295）

Ciclopirox Olamine（216，1258）

Ciclosporin（784）

Cilastatin Sodium（1253）

Cilnidipine（1302）

Cilostazol（754）

Cimetidine（142）

Cinametic Acid（1002）

Cinepazide Maleate（1293）

Cinmetacin（305）

Cinnarizine（306）

Ciprofibrate（783）

Ciprofloxacin（979）

Ciprofloxacin Hydrochloride（647，1100）

Ciprofloxacin Lactate（972）

Cisapride（753）

Cisplatin（297）

Citicoline（1000）

Citicoline Sodium（626，1096）

Citrate（1168）

Citric Acid（263，1239）

Clarithromycin（756）

Clavulanate Potassium（950）

Clebopride Malate（1058）

Clemastine Fumarate（514）

Clenbuterol Hydrochloride（351）

Clindamycin Hydrochloride（352）

Clindamycin Palmitate Hydrochloride（757）

Clindamycin Phosphate（614）

Clioquinol（506）

Clobetasol Propionate（592）

Clodronate Disodium（866，1219）

Clofazimine（671）

Clofibrate（494）

Clomifene Citrate（268）

Clomipramine Hydrochloride（842）

Clonazepam（502）

Clonidine Hydrochloride（327）

Cloperastine Hydrochloride（392）

Clopidogrel Bisulfate（1220）

Clorprenaline Hydrochloride（655）

Clotrimazole（169，1270）

Cloxacillin Sodium（200）

Clozapine（504）

Cobamamide（887）

Cocaine Hydrochloride（326）

Codeine（92）

Codeine Phosphate（577）

Coenzyme Q_{10}（1046）

Colchiceinamide（278）

Colchicine（277）

Colecalciferol（453）

Cortisone Acetate（544）

Crospovidone（937）

Crotamiton（951）

Cyanocobalamin（449）

Cyclandelate（217）

Cyclizine Hydrochloride（403）

Cycloclenbuterol Hydrochloride（362）

Cyclophosphamide（218）

Cypimegestrol Acetate（548）

Cyproheptadine Hydrochloride（404）

Cysteine（711）

Cysteine Hydrochloride（333，816）

Cystine（419，1036）

Cytarabine Hydrochloride（361）

D

D,L-α-Hydroxymethionine Calcium（1229）

Dacarbazine（1280）

Dactinomycin（177）

Daidzein（462）

Danazol（147）

Dapsone（412）

Daunorubicin Hydrochloride（323）

Decitabine（1232）

Decloxizine Hydrochloride（820）

Dehydrocholic Acid（715）

Deslanoside（74）

Dexamethasone（741）

Dexamethasone Acetate（546）

Dexamethasone Palmitate（1231）

Dexamethasone Sodium Phosphate（141）

Dexamfetamine（788）

Dexrazoxane（1317）

Dextromethorphan Hydrobromide（801）

Dextropropoxyphene Napsylate（1043）

Diatrizoic Acid（209）

Diazepam（138）

Diazoxide（1234）

Dibazol Hydrochloride（336）

Diclofenac Diethylamine（697）

Diclofenac Potassium（698）

Diclofenac Sodium（53）

Diclofenamide（54）

Didanosine（1294）

Diethylamine Salicylate（703）

Diethylcarbamazine Citrate（264）

Diethylstilbestrol（28）

Difenidol Hydrochloride（338）

Diflunisal（901）

Digoxin（139）

Dihydralazine Sulfate（482）

Dihydroartemisinin（696）

Dihydroetorphine Hydrochloride（313，1179）

Dihydrogalantamine（286）

Dihydroxyaluminium Aminoacetate（82）

Diisopropylamine Dichloroacetate（13）

Dilazep Hydrochloride（340）

Diltiazem Hydrochloride（337）

Dimenhydrinate（271）

Dimercaprol（15）

Dimercaptosuccinic Acid（14）

Dimethicone（10）

Dimethyl Ether（1109）

Dinatri Etidronas（1208）

L，L′-Dimethylcycleanine Dibromide（980）

Dioxopromethazine Hydrochloride（322）

Diphenhydramine Hydrochloride（365）

Diphenoxylate Hydrochloride（339）

Dipivefrine Hydrochloride（335）

Diprophylline（12）

Dipyridamole（557）

Disodium Edetate（978）

Disopyramide Phosphate（892）

Dithranol（140）

Dobutamine Hydrochloride（346）

Docetaxel（1136）

Domiphen Bromide（299）

Domperidone（606）

Donepezil Hydrochloride（1188）

Dopamine Hydrochloride（345）

Doxapram Hydrochloride（643，1256）

Doxazosin Mesilate（733）

Doxepin Hydrochloride（347）

Doxifluridine（716）

Doxofylline（941）

Doxorubicin Hydrochloride（1015）

Doxycycline Hydrochloride（386）

Ferrous Fumarate（513）

Ferrous Gluconate（879）

Ferrous Succinate（867）

Finasteride（793）

Flavoxate Hydrochloride（1031）

Fleroxacin（799）

Floctafenine（700）

Fluconazole（893）

Flucytosine（625）

Fludrocortisone Acetat（551）

Flumazenil（993）

Flunarizine Hydrochloride（379）

Fluocinolone Acetonide（800）

Fluorane（1312）

Fluocinolone Acetonide Acetate（550）

Fluorescein Sodium（273）

Fluorometholone（798）

Fluorouracil（280）

Fluoxetine Hydrochloride（837）

Fluphenazine Decanoate（279）

Fluphenazine Hydrochloride（378）

Flurazepam Hydrochloride（377）

Flurazepam Monohydrochloride（260）

Flurbiprofen（1169）

Flutamide（797）

Fluticasone Propionate（916）

Fluvastatin Sodium（1170）

Fluvoxamine Maleate（907）

Folic Acid（93）

Formylmerphalan（118）

Foscarnet Sodium（683）

Fosfomycin Calcium（1080）

Fosfomycin Sodium（1251）

Fosinopril Sodium（884）

Fructose Diphosphate（1297）

Ftibamzone（427）

Furapromide（179）

Furazabol（39，1146）

Furazolidone（182）

Furbenicillin Potassium（178）

Furosemide（184）

Fursultiamine（183）

G

Gabexate Mesilate（1131）

Gadodiamide（948）

Galactose（710）

Galantamine Hydrobromide（289）

Gallopamil Hydrochloride（815）

Ganciclovir（1266）

Gastrodin（914）

Gemcitabine Hydrochloride（1014）

Gemfibrozil（601）

Geniposide（992）

Gentamycin Sulfate（485）

Gestodene（724）

Gestrinone（925）

Glibenclamide（307）

Gliclazide（629）

Glimepiride（1085，1175）

Glipizide（808）

Gliquidone（630，1097）

Glucosamine Hydrochloride（652）

Glucose（464，702）

Glucurolactone（467）

Glutamic Acid（202，958，1263）

Glutamine（895）

L-Glutamine（201）

Glutathione（765）

Glutethimide（309）

Glycerol（77，1268）

Glycididazole Sodium（1129）

Glycine（81，929）

Glycopyrronium Bromide（308）

Glyfosfin（83）

Granisetron Hydrochloride（1027）

Griseofulvin（146）

Guacetisal（540，1276）

Guaifenesin（524）

Guanethidine Sulfate（667）

Guan-fu Base A Hydrochloride（645）

H

Halcinonide（498）

Halometasone（760）

Haloperidol（281）

Harringtonine（902）

Helicid（961）

Heparin Calcicum（203）

Heparin Sodium（204）

Hexestrol Bromoacetate（528）

Hexestrol Dipropionate（689）

Hexoprenaline Hydrochloride（383）

Histidine（785，981）

Histidine Hydrochloride（372）

Homatropine Hydrobromide（1172）

Homoharringtonine（420）

Huperzine A（936）

Hydralazine Hydrochloride（371）

Hydrobenzole Hydrochloride（388）

Hydrobromide（286）

Hydrochlorothiazide（285）

Hydrocortisone（283）

Hydrocortisone Acetate（552）

Hydrocortisone Butyrate（585）

Hydrocortisone Sodium Succinate（994）

Hydromorphone Hydrochloride（1321）

Hydroprednisone（284）

Hydroxycamptothecin（443）

Hydroxycarbamide（663）

Hydroxychloroquine Sulfate（490）

Hydroxymethylnicotinamide（439）

Hydroxyprogesterone Caproate（30）

Hydroxyurea（663）

Hymecromone（438）

Hypromellose Phthalate（1150）

I

Ibudilast（743）

Ibuprofen（85，943）

Idebenone（590，1134）

Idoxuridine（520）

Ifosfamide（1138）

Imidapril Hydrochloride（1024）

Imidazole Salicylate（589）

Imipenem（1254）

Imipramine Hydrochloride（638）

Imiquimod（1167）

Indapamide（192，1275）

Indobufen（1145）

Indocyanine Green（611）

Indomethacin（193）

Inosine（605）

Inositol（154）

Inositol Nicotinate（423）

Iohexol（1069）

Iopanoic Acid（522）

Iopromide（883，1070）

Iothalamic Acid（678）

Iotrolan（748）

Ioversol（882）

Ipriflavone（616，745）

Irbesartan（912）

Irsogladine Maleate（905）

D-Isocorydine Hydrochloride（1010）

Isoflurane（744，1139）

Isoleucine（165，894）

Isoniazid（166）

Isoprenaline Hydrochloride（349）

Isoproriram Fumarate（1211）

Isosorbide Dinitrate（473）

Isosorbide（1137）

Isosorbide Mononitrate（776）

Isotretinoin（944）

Isoxicam（151）

Isradipine（738）

Itopride Hydrochloride（1187）

Itraconazole（938）

J

Josamycin（1135）

Josamycin Propionate（1115）

K

Kanamycin Monosulfate（261）

Kanamycin Sulfate（484）

Ketamine Hydrochloride（393）

Ketoconazole（677）

α-Ketoleucine Calcium（1223）

α-Ketophenylalanine Calcium（1222）

Ketoprofen（517）

Ketorolac Tromethamine（1224）

Ketotifen Fumarate（515）

L

Lacidipine（976）

Lactose（256）

Lafutidine（1160）

Lamivudine（975）

Lamotrigine（780）

Lansoprazole（708）

Lappaconitine Hydrobromide（290）

Latamoxef Sodium（1161）

Laurocapram（48）

Leflunomide（954）

Letrozol（953）

Leucine（298，987）

Leucogen（955）

Levamisole Hydrochloride（325）

Levobunolol Hydrochloride（636）

Levocarnitine（591）

Levodopa（87）

Levofloxacin（1128）

Levofloxacin Hydrochloride（1012）

Levofloxacin Lactate（970）

Levofloxacin Mesylate（1132）

Levoglutamide（201）

Levonorgestrel（726）

Levothyroxine Sodium（928）

Lidocaine Hydrochloride（357）

Ligustrazine Hydrochloride（319，1098）

Ligustrazine Phosphate（1259）

Lincomycin Hydrochloride（833）

Lindane（977）

Liranaftate（1298）

Lisinopril（676）

Lobeline Hydrochloride（318，1197）

Lobenzarit Sodium（670）

Lodoxamide Tromethamine（803）

Lofexidine Hydrochloride（1025）

Lomefloxacin Hydrochloride（650）

Lomustine（300）

Loperamide Hydrochloride（649，1257）

Loratadine（865）

Lorazepam（1144）

Losartan Potassium（764）

Lovastatin（802）

Loxapine Succinate（686）

Loxoprofen Sodium（995）

Lysine（1071）

Lysine Acetate（890）

Lysine Hydrochloride（399，1035）

M

Mafenide Acetate（556）

Magnesium Salicylate（60）

Magnesium Valproate（66，1114）

Malotilate（34）

Mandelic Acid（989）

Mannitol（84，1238）

Maprotiline Hydrochloride（634）

Matrine（982）

Mazindol（691）

Mebendazole（Polymorph A）（100）

Mebendazole（Polymorph C）（101）

Meclofenamic Acid（116）

Meclofenoxate Hydrochloride（331）

Mecobalamin（732）

Medroxyprogesterone Acetate（160）

Mefenamic Acid（730）

Megestrol Acetate（545）

Meglumine（463）

Meglumine Gadopentetate（736）

Meloxicam（998）

Menadiol Diacetate（458）

Menadione Sodium Bisulfite（457）

Menthol（891）

Mephedrine Hydrochloride（330）

Mephentermine Sulfate（489）

Mepixanox（731）

Meprobamate（99）

Mercaptopurine（516）

Meropenem（997）

Mesalazine（996）

Mesna（1174）

Metacycline（111）

Metacycline Hydrochloride（1026）

Metamizole Sodium（159）

Metaraminol Bitartrate（294，1262）

Metformin Hydrochloride（631）

Methaqualone（115）

Methazolamide（1077）

Methenamine（45）

Methionine（444，1045）

Methocarbamol（303）

Methotrexate（108）

Methoxamine Hydrochloride（329）

Methoxsalen（105）

Methoxyflurane（106）

Methoxymerphalan（104）

Methoxyphenamine Hydrochloride（1086）

Methybenactyzium Bromide（680）

Methyl Salicylate（709）

Methylcantharidinimide（931）

Methyldopa（930）

Methylindirubin（595）

Methylparaben（853）

Methylphenidate Hydrochloride（374）

Methylprednisolone Hemisuccinate（1060）

Methyltestosterone（120）

Methylthioninum Chloride（143）

Methylthiouracil（114）

Metildigoxin（728）

Metoclopramide（107）

Metoprolol（685）

Metoprolol Tartrate（425）

Metronidazole（112）

Metronidazole Benzoate（113）

Mexiletine Hydrochloride（381）

Mezlocillin Sodium（627）

Mianserin Hydrochloride（1191）

Miconazole（276）

Miconazole Nitrate（474）

Micronomicin Sulfate（479）

Midazolam（1084）

Mifepristone（162，896，1141）

Milrinone（749）

Minocycline Hydrochloride（825）

Minoxidil（608）

Mitiglinide Calcium（1243）

Mitobronitol（16）

Mitomycin（918）

Mitoxantrone Hydrochloride（824）

Mizolastine（1166）

Moclobemide（740）

Molsidomine（1240）

Mometasone Furoate（814）

Monoclofenamic Acid（497）

Montelukast Sodium（1242）

Moracizine Hydrochloride（651）

Moroxydine Hydrochloride（343）

Morphine（739）

Morphine Hydrochloride（344）

Morphine Sulfate（873）

Mosapride Citrate（991）

Moxifloxacin Hydrochloride（1319）

Moxonidine Hydrochloride（1029）

Mupirocin（845）

Mupirocin Lithium（844）

Mycophenolate Mofetil（1241）

N

Nabumetone（661）

Nadifloxacin（1300）

Nafcillin Sodium（1322）

Naftifine Hydrochloride（1030）

Naftopidil（1042）

Nalidixic Acid（431）

Nalorphine Hydrobromide（291）

Naloxone Hydrochloride（646）

Naltrexone Hydrochloride（1194）

Nandrolone Phenylpropionate（231）

Naphazoline Hydrochloride（385）

Naphthoquine（662）

Naphthoquine Phosphate（734）

α-Naphthylacetic Acid（855）

Naproxen（432）

Naproxen Sodium（433）

Nateglinide（1142）

Nefopam Hydrochloride（367）

Nemonapride（856）

Neoandrographolide（302）

Neomycin Sulfate（492）

Neostigmine Bromide（526）

Neostigmine Methylsulfate（110）

Nevirapine（1159）

Nicardipine Hydrochloride（334）

Nicergoline（926）

Niclosamide（503）

Nicorandil（134）

Nicotinamide（421）

Nicotinic Acid（422）

Nicotinylmethylamide（439）

Nifedipine（469）

Nifuratel（868）

Nikethamide（135）

Nilestriol（136）

Nimesulide（598）

Nimodipine（599）

Nimustine Hydrochloride（1301）

Nisoldipine（927，1127）

Nitrazepam（470）

Nitrendipine（600）

Nitrofural（180）

Nitrofurantoin（181）

Nitrofurazone（180）

Nonoxinol（43）

Noradrenaline Bitartrate（293）

Norcantharidin（920，1309）

Norethisterone（258）

Norethisterone Enanthate （779）

Norfloxacin Glutamate （960）

Norfloxacin Lactate （1154）

Norfloxacin （1202）

Norgestrel （109）

Norpseudoephedrine Hydrochloride （818）

Noscapine （609）

O

Ofloxacin （1003）

Olanzapine （1210）

Oleanolic Acid （158，1091）

Olmesartan Medoxomil （1306）

Olprinone Hydrochloride （1246）

Olsalazine Disodium （858）

Omeprazole （675，1050）

Omeprazole Sodium （1051）

Ondansetron Hydrochloride （832）

Orazamide （1049）

Ornidazole （1052）

Oxacillin Sodium （239）

Oxaliplatin （1209）

Oxantel Pamoate （1286）

Oxaprozin （679）

Oxazepam （75）

Oxiracetam （1063）

Oxybuprocaine Hydrochloride （316）

Oxybutynin Hydrochloride （1032）

Oxyfedrine Hydrochloride （394）

Oxymetazoline Hydrochloride （653）

Oxyphenbutazone （440）

Oxytetracycline （24）

Oxytetracycline Hydrochloride （1064）

Ozagrel （674）

Ozagrel Sodium （1048）

P

Paclitaxel （875）

Paeoniflorin （752）

Paeonol （46）

Palmitic Acid （862）

Pamidronate Disodium （778）

Pantoprazole Sodium （1083）

Papaverine Hydrochloride （405）

Paracetamol （131）

Pargyline Hydrochloride （1313）

Paromomycin Sulfate （483）

Paroxetine Hydrochloride （831）

Pefloxacin Mesylate （933）

Penciclovir （1047）

Penehyclidine Hydrochloride （1186）

Penfluridol （41）

Penicillamine （224）

Pentetrazol （727）

Pentoxifylline （29）

Pentoxyverine Citrate （267）

Pergolide Mesilate （735）

Perindopril Erbumine （1204）

Perindopril （847）

Perphenazine （243）

Pethidine Hydrochloride （376）

Phanquinone （207）

Phenacetin （247）

Phenazone （161）

Phencynonate Hydrochloride （1021）

Phenformin Hydrochloride （363）

Phenobarbital （227）

Phenobarbital Sodium （228）

Phenol （240）

Phenolphthalein （429）

Phenoxybenzamine Hydrochloride （384）

Phenoxymethylpenicillin Potassium （792）

Phenprobamate （229）

Phentolamine Hydrochloride （353）

Phentolamine Mesylate （121）

Phenylalanine（230，983）

Phenylbutazone（296）

Phenylephrine Hydrochloride（819）

Phenylpropanol（232）

Phenylpropanolamine Hydrochloride（364）

Phenytoin Sodium（238）

Pholcodine（531）

Phthalylsulfathiazole（428）

Phtiobuzone（427）

Physostigmine Salicylate（58）

Phytomenadione（456）

Pidotimod（693）

Pilocarpine Nitrate（472）

Pinacidil（762）

Pinaverium Bromide（694）

Pindolol（610）

Pinitol（225）

Pioglitazone Hydrochloride（1192）

Pipemidic Acid（189）

Piperacetamide（8）

Piperacillin（621）

Piperacillin Sodium（407）

Piperaquine（274）

Piperaquine Phosphate（580）

Piperazine Ferulate（969）

Piperazine Phosphate（581）

Pipotiazine Palmitate（622）

Piracetam（185）

Pirenoxine（763）

Pirenoxine Sodium（187）

Pirenzepine Hydrochloride（648）

Pirfenoxone Sodium（187）

Piribedil（761）

Piroxicam（188）

Pizotifen（242）

Podophyllotoxin（805）

Poloxamer（618）

Potassium Sorbate（688）

Pralidoxime Chloride（1218）

Pralidoxime Iodide（523）

Pranlukast（1212）

Pravastatin Sodium（860）

Praziquantel（190）

Prazosin Hydrochloride（375）

Prednisolone（284）

Prednisolone Acetate（553）

Prednisone（612，782）

Prednisone Acetate（549）

Pregnenolone Acetylsalicylate（6）

Prenylamine Lactate（255）

Primaquine Phosphate（578）

Primidone（62）

Probenecid（73）

Probucol（1054）

Procainamide Hydrochloride（398）

Procaine Benzylpenicillin（511）

Procaine Hydrochloride（397）

Procaterol Hydrochloride（637）

Progesterone（434）

Proglumide（67）

Proline（436，1041）

Prolonium Iodide（512）

Promethazine Hydrochloride（350）

Propafenone Hydrochloride（395）

Propantheline Bromide（525）

Propiverine Hydrochloride（1009）

Propofol（707）

Propranolol Hydrochloride（396）

Propyl Gallate（1038）

Propylene Glycol（706）

Propylparaben（852）

Propylthiouracil（70）

Propyphenazone（942）

Protionamide（69）

Protirelin（1055）

Pseudoephedrine（604）

Pseudoephedrine Hydrochloride（642）

Pseudoephedrine Sulfate（1062）

Puerarin（878）

Pyrantel Pamoate（51）

Pyrazinamide（191）

Pyricarbate（186）

Pyridostigmine Bromide（527）

Pyridoxine Hydrochloride（448）

Pyrimethamine（3）

Pyrithione Sodium（1272）

Pyritinol Hydrochloride（356）

Pyronaride（684）

Pyrozoline（435）

Q

Quetiapine Fumarate（1053，1273）

Quinapril Hydrochloride（1200）

Quinestrol（1163）

Quinine Dihydrochloride（11）

Quinine Hydrochloride（373，1101）

Quinine Sulfate（488）

R

Raceanisodamine（811）

Racecadotril（1005）

Ramipril（1074）

Ramosetron Hydrochloride（1311）

Ranitidine Hydrochloride（401）

Raubasine（1044）

Rebamipide（1067）

Remamlate Hydrochloride（400）

Remifentanil Hydrochloride（1288）

Repaglinide（1068）

Reserpine（195）

Resorcinol（206）

Resormelate Hydrochloride（400）

Retinamide Acid（849）

Retinol Acetate（446）

Rhapontin（23）

Ribavirin（22）

Riboflavin（447）

Riboflavin Sodium Phosphate（628）

Riboflavin Tetrabutyrate（310）

Rifabutin（1250）

Rifampicin（198）

Rifandine（952）

Rifapentine（199，1143）

Rimantadine Hydrochloride（1196）

Rimexolone（758）

Risperidone（759）

Rorifone（532）

Rosiglitazone Maleate（906）

Rotundine（251）

Rosuvastatin Calcium（1244）

Rotundine Hydrochloride（834）

Roxatidine Acetate Hydrochloride（1248）

Roxithromycin（786）

Rubidate（269）

Rufluoxacin Hydrochloride（827）

Rupatadine Fumarate（1237）

Rutin（174）

S

Saccharin Sodium（576）

Salbutamol Sulfate（486）

Salicylic Acid（57）

Salmeterol Xinafoate（1162）

Scopolamine Butylbromide（21）

Scopolamine Hydrobromide（288）

Secobarbital Sodium（137）

Securinine Nitrate（471）

Selegiline Hydrochloride（821）

Semustine（1119）

Serine（133，917）

Sertraline Hydrochloride（835）

Sevoflurane（1108）

Sibutramine Hydrochloride（1016）

Sildenafil Citrate（990）

Silymarin（56）

Simvastatin（962）

Sinomenine Hydrochloride（1023）

Sodium Aminosalicylate（132）

Sodium Ascorbate（1039）

Sodium Benzoate（234）

Sodium Camphorsulfonate（537）

Sodium Cromoglycate（155）

Sodium Cyclamate（669）

Sodium Dimercaptosuccinate（1281）

Sodium Etacrynate（197）

Sodium Ferulate（775）

Sodium Fusidate（1235）

Sodium Glutamate（959）

Sodium Glycerophosphate（79）

Sodium Houttuyfonate（153）

Sodium Hyaluronate（1173）

Sodium Hydroxybutyrate（437）

Sodium Hydroxypropylcromate（157）

Sodium Ibandronate（939）

Sodium Nitroprusside（1061）

Sodium Oxybate（437）

Sodium Paeonolsilate（47）

Sodium Prasterone Sulfate（874）

Sodium Salicylate（59）

Sodium Valproate（65）

Solaziquone（144）

Sorbic Acid（25）

Sorbitol（26，1278）

Sotalol Hydrochloride（1028，1199）

Sparfloxacin（921）

Spectinomycin Hydrochloride（1007）

Spironolactone（582）

Squalene（205）

Stanozolol（597）

Stigmasterol（766）

Streptomycin Sulfate（491）

Strophanthin K（262）

Strychnine Nitrate（869）

Sufentanil Citrate（1320）

Sulbactam Sodium（509）

Sulbenicillin（1228）

Sulfacetamide Sodiurn（574）

Sulfadiazine（570）

Sulfadiazine Silver（572）

Sulfadiazine Sodium（571）

Sulfadiazine Zinc（573）

Sulfadimidine（562）

Sulfadoxine（567）

Sulfafurazole（561）

Sulfaguanidine（569）

Sulfalene（563）

Sulfamethoxazole（565）

Sulfamethoxydiazine（566）

Sulfamethoxypyridazine（564）

Sulfamonomethoxine（568）

Sulfanilamide（560）

Sulfasalazine（620）

Sulfobromophthalein Sodium（575）

Sulindac（877）

Sulpiride（510）

Sultamicillin Mesylate（934）

Sultamicillin Tosilate（1261）

Sultopride Hydrochloride（1282）

Sumatriptan（876）

Suxamethonium Chloride（496）

Synephrine Tartrate（846）

T

Tamoxifen Citrate（265）

Tamsulosin Hydrochloride（830）

Taurine（44）

Tazarotene（919，1116）

Tazobactam（1260）

Tegadifur（52）

Tegafur（861）

Tegaserod Maleate（1111）

Teicoplanin（1214）

Telbivudine（1213）

Telmisartan（1057）

Temozolomide（1216）

Teniposide（1056）

Terazosin Hydrochloride（841）

Terbinafine Hydrochloride（840，1198）

Terbutaline Sulfate（668）

Terfenadine（244）

Testosterone Propionate（72）

Testosterone Undecanoate（584）

Tetra（2-Methoxy Isobutyl Isonitrile）Copper（I）
  Boroflueride（717）

Tetracaine Hydrochloride（314）

Tetracycline（122）

Tetracycline Hydrochloride（332）

Tetrandrine Dimethiodide（123）

Thalidomide（1149）

Theobromine（91）

Theophylline（272）

Thiamazole（117）

Thiamine Hydrochloride（654）

Thiamine Nitrate（476）

Thiamphenicol Glycinate Hydrochloride（1247）

Thiamphenicol（594）

Thiocolchicoside（870）

Thiopental Sodium（871）

Thioridazine Hydrochloride（1034）

Thiotipa（530）

Threonine（175，957）

Thymol（767）

Thyroxine（729）

Tiabendazole（1316）

Tiabendazole（1316）

Tiapride Hydrochloride（1033）

Tibolone（1215）

Ticlopidine Hydrochloride（640）

Timolol Maleate（33）

Timonacic（682）

Tinidazole（665）

Tioguanine（477）

Tiopronin（872）

Tiotropium Bromide（1078）

Tocopherol Acetate（455）

Tocopherol Nicotinate（454）

Tolazoline Hydrochloride（1193）

Tolbutamide（102）

Tolmetin Sodium（945）

Tolperisone Hydrochloride（342，1099）

Tolterodine Tartrate（1037）

Topiramate（949）

Topotecan Hydrochloride（1020）

Toremifene Citrate（795）

Tosufloxacin Tosilate（932）

Tramadol Hydrochloride（641）

Tranexamic Acid（409）

Tranilast（150，1140）

Trapidil（149）

Trepibutone（148）

Tretinoin（445）

Triamcinolone（747）

Triamcinolone Acetonide（603）

Triamcinolone Acetonide Acetate（547）

Triamterene（413）

Triazolam（586）

Tribendimidine（1295）

Trifluperazine Hydrochloride（317）

Trihexyphenidyl Hydrochloride（366）

Trimebutine Maleate（725）

Trimetazidine Hydrochloride（1189）

Trimethoprim（103）

Triprolidine Hydrochloride（1190）

Triptolide（1073）

Trometamol（408）

Tropicamide（746，1267）

Troxipide（1277）

Tryptophan（156，946）

Tulobuterol Hydrochloride（358）

Tyrosine（518，1072）

U

Ubenimex（911）

Ubidecarenone（1082）

Ufenamate（623）

Ulinastatin（909）

Undecylenic Acid（17）

Urapidil（910）

Urapidil Hydrochloride（1181）

Urea（210）

Ursodeoxycholic Acid（534）

V

Valacyclovir Hydrochloride（1013）

Valine（559，1076）

Valproate Semisodium（1252）

Valpromide（64）

Valsartan（1227）

Vancomycin（1180）

Vanillin（1001）

Vecuronium Bromide（848）

Venlafaxine Hydrochloride（1008，1265）

Verapamil Hydrochloride（389）

Viaminate（1207）

Vidarabine（968）

Vidarabine Monophosphate（777）

Vidarabine Phosphate（1093）

Vigabatrin（810）

Vinblastine Sulfate（481）

Vincamine（705）

Vincristine Sulfate（480）

Vindesine Sulfate（1299）

Vinorelbine Tartrate（1315）

Vinpocetine（588）

Vitamin A Acetate（446）

Vitamin B_1（1205）

Vitamin B_2（447）

Vitamin B_6（448）

Vitamin B_{12}（449）

Vitamin C（450）

Vitamin D_2（452）

Vitamin D_3（453）

Vitamin E（1206）

Vitamin E Acetate（455）

Vitamin E Nicotinate（454）

Vitamin K_1（456）

Vitamin K_4（458）

Vitamin U（459）

Voglibose（940）

W

Warfarin Sodium（152）

X

Xantinol Nicotinate（660）

Xylitol（40，1088）

Xylometazoline Hydrochloride（657，1279）

Z

Zinc Acexamate（583，888，1103）

Zinc Gluconate（466）

Zinc Undecylenate（18）

Zolpidem Tartrate（1203）

Zopiclone（755）